Understanding
Health Inequalities

Second Edition

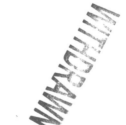

Understanding Health Inequalities

Second Edition

Edited by Hilary Graham

 Open University Press

Open University Press
McGraw-Hill Education
McGraw-Hill House
Shoppenhangers Road
Maidenhead
Berkshire
England
SL6 2QL

email: enquiries@openup.co.uk
world wide web: www.openup.co.uk

and Two Penn Plaza, New York, NY 10121-2289, USA

First published 2009
Reprinted 2010

Copyright © Hilary Graham 2009

A catalogue record of this book is available from the British Library

ISBN10: 0 335 23459 3 (pb)
ISBN13: 978 0 335 23459 2 (pb)

Library of Congress Cataloging-in-Publication Data
CIP data has been applied for

Fictitous names of companies, products, people, characters and/or data that may be used herein (in case studies or in examples) are not intended to represent any real individual, company, product or event.

Typeset by Aptara Inc., India
Printed in the UK by CPI Antony Rowe, Chippenham, Wiltshire

The **McGraw·Hill** Companies

Contents

Part 1: Health inequalities: understanding patterns over time and place

Part 2: Health inequalities: understanding intersections

Part 3: Health inequalities: understanding policy impacts

List of contributors

Karl Atkin, Senior Lecturer, Department of Health Sciences, University of York.

Mel Bartley, Professor of Medical Sociology, Department of Epidemiology and Public Health, University College London.

G. David Batty, Wellcome Trust Research Fellow, MRC Social and Public Health Sciences Unit, University of Glasgow.

David Blane, Professor of Medical Sociology, Division of Epidemiology, Public Health and Primary Care, Imperial College London.

Bo Burström, Professor in Social Medicine, Department of Public Health Sciences, Karolinska Institute, Stockholm.

Danny Dorling, Professor of Human Geography, Social and Spatial Inequalities Group, Department of Geography, University of Sheffield.

Anne Ellaway, Senior Research Scientist, MRC Social and Public Health Sciences Unit, University of Glasgow.

Hilary Graham, Professor of Health Sciences, Department of Health Sciences, University of York.

Barbara Hanratty, Senior Lecturer in Population and Community Health, Division of Public Health, University of Liverpool.

Kate Hunt, Professor and Head of Gender and Health Programme, MRC Social and Public Health Sciences Unit, University of Glasgow.

Saffron Karlsen, Senior Research Fellow, Department of Epidemiology and Public Health, University College London.

Catherine Law, Professor of Public Health and Epidemiology, Centre for Paediatric Epidemiology and Biostatistics, UCL Institute of Child Health, London.

Sally Macintyre, Professor of Social and Public Health Science, University of Glasgow, and Honorary Director, MRC Social and Public Health Sciences Unit.

James Nazroo, Professor of Sociology, School of Social Sciences, University of Manchester.

Naomi Rudoe, Research Student, Faculty of Education and Language Studies, The Open University.

Bethan Thomas, Researcher, Social and Spatial Inequalities Group, Department of Geography, University of Sheffield.

Rachel Thomson, Professor of Social Research, Faculty of Health and Social Care, The Open University.

Margaret Whitehead, WH Duncan Professor of Public Health, Division of Public Health, University of Liverpool.

Acknowledgements

This new edition of *Understanding Health Inequalities* presents 11 new chapters by authors at the forefront of research on social and health inequalities. It includes authors who contributed to the first edition of the book published in 2000. The book's authorship has also been extended for the new edition to give emphasis to the intersections between socio-economic inequality and other dimensions of inequality and identity, including age, gender, ethnicity and religion.

I would like to thank Sally Stephenson, University of York, for her help with the preparation of the manuscript.

Hilary Graham

List of tables and figures

Figures

Tables

Box

Introduction: the challenge of health inequalities

Hilary Graham

Introduction

The opportunity to live a long and healthy life remains profoundly unequal. In both childhood and adulthood, social disadvantage is associated with a higher risk of disease, disability and premature death. But it is not only the poorest groups whose health is compromised by their socio-economic circumstances. The link between poor circumstances and poor health is part of a broader association between people's socio-economic position and their health. It is part of a social gradient in which those on the middle rungs of the socio-economic ladder enjoy better health and live longer lives than those in the most disadvantaged circumstances, but fail to reach the health standards achieved by the most advantaged groups.

This social gradient in health has endured over time, across societies and despite changes in the major causes of death. Thus, it is evident in low-income societies where infectious diseases keep death rates high and many children die in infancy – and in rich societies where death rates are low, chronic disease predominates and deaths are concentrated in older age groups. These socio-economic inequalities in health have persisted despite marked improvements both in living standards and in health in most regions of the world. Global recession is exerting a downward drag on life chances and living standards, with those already in poorer circumstances bearing the brunt (OECD, 2008). A worsening economic climate makes it imperative that we understand how people's circumstances affect their health.

Understanding health inequalities is the aim of the book. It seeks to provide an accessible overview of mechanisms underlying the association between socio-economic position and health. Chapters explore life-course pathways, explaining how exposure to disadvantage takes its toll on health from early life and into adulthood, and investigate how the areas in which we live influence our chances of leading a long and healthy life. Woven through the book is a concern with how other dimensions of inequality, like ethnicity and gender, intersect with socio-economic position in making a difference to people's lives and to their health. Thus, the book includes chapters which turn the spotlight on ethnic, religious and cultural factors and on the intersections between gender and socio-economic position. The impact of policy on inequalities in health is also a theme running through the book, and is explicitly addressed in the final chapters.

In the quest to deepen understanding of health inequalities, the chapters draw particularly on research from the United Kingdom (UK). The UK provides an illuminating case study. First, it exhibits trends evident in other high-income societies, where, as in the UK, greater prosperity and better overall health have been achieved without a narrowing of health inequalities. Second, the UK's long tradition of research on health inequalities means that it has a rich data infrastructure through which to investigate their causes. The book draws on cross-sectional studies, where individuals are surveyed at one point in time, and longitudinal studies following individuals over time, often from birth and across long periods of their lives. It draws, too, on qualitative studies, where people talk in their own terms about how they understand their place in society, their lives and their health. To exploit these data sources, the book brings epidemiologists, sociologists, geographers and policy analysts together with researchers with a background in gender and ethnic studies.

This introductory chapter sets the scene for the book. It includes a brief discussion of the concept of health inequalities and the measures used to capture the social patterning of health. The chapter then presents evidence on socio-economic inequalities in health and discusses the ways in which research has sought to explain them. It concludes by introducing the chapters and outlining their contribution to understanding health inequalities.

What are health inequalities?

People in poor health are not randomly distributed across the population. Instead, they tend to be concentrated among those with fewer of the resources which enable people to live economically secure and prosperous lives. As an example, Figure 1 maps the patterning of health across income groups in England, charting the proportion of men and women who rate their health as 'not good' (that is, as fair, bad or very bad as opposed to good or very good). As it indicates, the proportion increases from around 15 per cent in the richest fifth of households to around 40 per cent in the poorest fifth of households (Sproston and Primatesta, 2004). The patterns captured for men and women in Figure 1 are found not only among the majority white population. They are evident, too, among the UK's

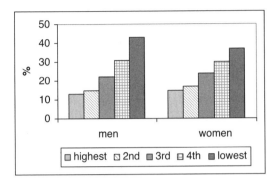

Figure 1 Proportion of women and men aged 16 and over assessing their health as 'not good' (as fair, bad or very bad) by income quintile based on equivalized household income, England, 2003.
Source: Sproston and Primatesta (2004), Table 10.3.

minority ethnic groups. Figure 2 captures patterns among some of these groups.

The patterns described in Figures 1 and 2 are referred to as 'health inequalities'. The term captures the fact that there are systematic differences in the health of people occupying unequal positions in society. It is used to refer to health differences associated with people's unequal socioeconomic position as well as health inequalities between ethnic groups and between men and women. The later dimensions tend to be explicitly labelled as 'ethnic inequalities in health' and 'gender inequalities in health'.

While widely used by the research and policy communities, 'health inequalities' does not have universal currency. In the United States (USA) for example, researchers and policy makers rarely talk of health inequalities when describing the systematic health differences between more and less advantaged groups. They use 'health disparities' instead. In the UK, the Conservative governments of the 1980s and 1990s dropped references to heath inequalities in favour of 'health variations'; health inequalities re-entered the political vernacular with the election of the Labour government in 1997. Terms like 'variations' and 'disparities' tend to be preferred by scientific and political constituencies willing to acknowledge health differences between population sub-groups – but who are uncomfortable with concepts that draw explicit attention to the societal inequalities to which these health differences are linked.

Whether 'health inequalities' or 'health disparities' is preferred, it is typically used descriptively to capture the fact that social differences between people are associated with health differences between them (as

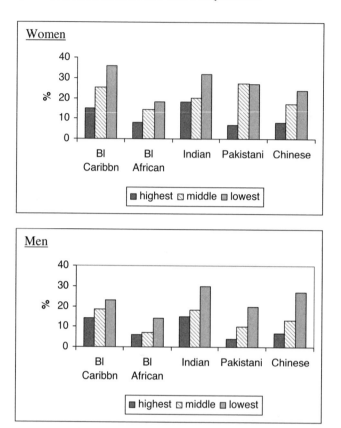

Figure 2 Proportion of men and women aged 16 and over assessing their health as 'not good' (as fair, bad or very bad) within ethnic minority groups by income tertile based on equivalised household income, England 2004. *Source:* Sproston and Mindell (2006), Table 2.4.

Figures 1 and 2 illustrate). 'Health inequities' is often used when commentators wish to convey a moral judgement about this social patterning. As Whitehead and Dahlgren (2007: 3) put it, 'social inequities are differences widely considered to be unfair'. The commonly held view that children should have an equal chance of living a long and healthy life means that inequalities in children's health are widely regarded as inequitable. More broadly, health inequalities are defined as health inequities by those who believe that everyone should have the opportunity to achieve the standards of health enjoyed by those in the most advantaged circumstances.

Researching socio-economic inequalities in health

While there is a considerable amount of evidence on health inequalities, it is limited in important ways. First, the evidence comes predominantly from rich countries in which only a minority of the world's population lives. In part, this is because these countries have more comprehensive data collection systems. In England and Wales, national registration systems for births and deaths have been in place since the early 19th century. Two centuries on, the functioning vital registration systems required to measure life expectancy are estimated to cover only 1 in 3 deaths worldwide (Lopez et al., 2001). Deficiencies in the data infrastructure of poorer countries reflect a wider pattern of unequal investment in health research. It is estimated that 90 per cent of global health research funding is spent on the richest 10 per cent of the world's population who already enjoy the highest standards of health.

Further, research on health inequalities has traditionally focused on some rather than all population sub-groups, with much of the evidence coming from studies of men, and white men in particular (Pollitt et al., 2005). In consequence, considerably less is known about the socio-economic patterning of health among women and between women and men (see Chapter 2.3) and about how ethnic and cultural differences influence people's health (see Chapters 2.1 and 2.2). Much less is known, too, about how multiple dimensions of social inequality – socio-economic position, gender and ethnicity for example – combine to shape people's life chances and their health (explored in Chapters 2.1 to 2.4).

Second, the evidence consists largely of data on individuals, gleaned from official records and from cross-sectional and longitudinal surveys. These individual data shed light on the links between people's socio-economic circumstances – as measured for example by their occupation or household income – and their health. The data have therefore enabled researchers to trace the influence of childhood circumstances on adult health, and to identify the role of intermediary factors, like material conditions and health behaviours. However, individual-level data tell us relatively little about the wider social forces which produce inequalities in people's lives. Our lives are regulated by an intricate web of social institutions, including the education system, the labour market and the welfare state, and we are continually stratified as we make our way through them – yet these stratifying processes are hard to capture in data collected on individuals (Graham, 2007). With little information on the operation of the wider society, health inequalities research has been slow to recognize how prejudice and discrimination can impact on people's lives and can influence their health. Chapters 2.1 and 2.2 set the health experiences of religious and ethnic minorities in this wider context, while Chapter 2.4 draws on qualitative studies of young people to challenge social stereotypes of teenage mothers.

While individual-level data shed only a partial light on the wider social structure, they tell us considerably more about people's position within it. They tell us about an individual's educational level, occupational status and income for example. These are important pieces of information. In the UK, as in other rich societies, educational qualifications are increasingly needed to gain entry to the labour market and, particularly, to obtain well-paid and secure jobs. Income from paid work, in the form of wages, salaries and occupational pensions, underwrites the living standards of most households. Education, occupation and income are therefore regarded as both core constituents and key measures of socio-economic position. Finely graded information can be collected on these dimensions; for example, from no educational qualifications to degree-level qualifications, from low-skilled manual work to high-skilled non-manual work and from low income to high income. Residential patterns tend to vary in line with socio-economic position, with richer people tending to live in areas with a high proportion of rich people while poorer people are over-represented in neighbourhoods where incomes are low. This means that people's socio-economic circumstances can be measured using indicators of the areas in which they live. These different measures of socio-economic position are discussed briefly in turn.

Measures of people's socio-economic circumstances

Education is the principal measure of socio-economic position in the majority of high-income countries, including the USA and most of Europe. Indicators like highest educational attainment and years of full-time education are inclusive measures (almost everyone goes to school) which, in contrast to occupation or income, change little across adulthood. Further, because educational level is typically set by early adulthood, it provides a measure of socio-economic position which is independent of subsequent health status. This is particularly important for studies seeking to establish the contribution of socio-economic disadvantage to future health.

However, there are some limitations. Education level is ambiguously placed between childhood socio-economic circumstances – which influence how long young people stay in full-time education and how well they do at exams – and future adult socio-economic position – which is influenced by their success in the education system. Further, because governments set the age of leaving full-time education and determine the structure of qualifications, changes in educational policy can produce marked changes in the socio-economic profile of the population. For example in Britain in the 1940s, 90 per cent of women fell into the lowest educational category, with no secondary education and no educational qualifications (Douglas and Blomfield, 1958). Today, full-time secondary education to the age of 16 is required for all young people and a third of young women can expect to secure the qualifications they need to enter higher education (Machin, 2003). As these dramatic changes indicate, education-based measures of socio-economic position need to be used with caution in analyses investigating health inequalities across age groups and over time.

Occupation is the dominant measure of socio-economic position (or social class as it has traditionally been called) in the UK. Children have been conventionally classified by their father's occupation (or mother if he is not present in the household) and, while widely criticized, partner's occupation is often used for women living with men. An early classification divided the population into 'three great classes' consisting of 'the gentry and professional people and their families', 'farmers and tradesmen and their families' and 'artisans, labourers and their families'. The classification captured the pecking order of power and prestige in 19th-century Britain, a pecking order in which women and children earned their social class indirectly through the occupation of 'the man of the house'. The social gradients in health which the schema revealed are presented in Figure 3.

The social class schema was extended and formalized in a classification developed by the Registrar General at the beginning of the 20th century. By the 1920s, it had evolved into a five-fold division of occupational classes which became the official measure of socio-economic position in the UK until 2000. Described in Table 1, the classification is used in this chapter (Figures 4 and 5) and Chapter 1.2.

In 2001, a new system for measuring socio-economic position replaced the 100-year old Registrar General's schema as the UK's official classification. The National Statistics-Socioeconomic Classification (NS-SEC) places occupations into groups on the basis of their dominant employment relations and conditions, such as whether wages or salaries are paid, how much job security and autonomy workers have, and whether there is a career structure and prospects for promotion (Rose and Pevalin, 2003). Table 2 describes two simplified typologies which can be derived from the classification (the five-category version is used in Chapters 1.1 and 2.3; the three-category version in Figure 7). The three-category NS-SEC also provides the basis of England's health inequality target for infant mortality set by the government to be met by 2010 (see Chapter 1.3). The target focuses on infants for whom information on father's occupation is recorded on their birth certificates. It seeks to reduce the gap in mortality rates between infants born to fathers with occupations in the 'routine and manual'

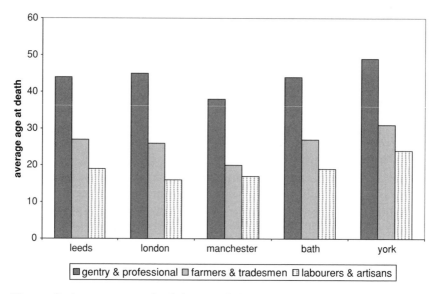

Figure 3 Average age at death by social class: Leeds, London (Bethnal Green), Manchester, Bath and York, 1838–41.
Source: adapted from Lancet (1843); Royal Commission on the Health of Towns (1845).

socio-economic group and all children in England who can be allocated to a socio-economic group. However, occupational information is currently only collected for fathers who are either married to the mother or register the birth with her. Babies solely registered by mothers therefore fall outside the target group. While they represent a relatively small group (7% of all live births), they have higher infant mortality rates than babies born to fathers in the routine and manual group (6.5 compared with 5.6 deaths

Table 1   Registrar General's social class classification

Social class		Examples of occupations
I	Professional occupations	Doctor, accountant
II	Managerial and intermediate occupations	Teacher, manager
III	Skilled occupations	
	NM: non-manual	Secretary, sales representative
	M: manual	Bus driver, electrician
IV	Partly skilled occupations	Security guard, assembly worker
V	Unskilled occupations	Office cleaner, labourer

Table 2 National Statistics-Socioeconomic Classification (NS-SEC): five-class and three-class versions

Five classes	*Three classes*
1 Managerial and professional occupations	1 Managerial and professional occupations
2 Intermediate occupations	2 Intermediate occupations
3 Small employers and own-account workers	3 Routine and manual occupations
4 Lower supervisory and technical occupations	
5 Semi-routine and routine occupations	
Never worked and long-term unemployed	Never worked and long-term unemployed

Source: Rose and Pevalin (2003), Figure 1.3.

per 1000 live births in 2004–06) (DH[formerly DoH], 2008). The UK is currently amending the regulations regarding the registration of births to require mothers to include details of the father, including his occupation, except in specified circumstances (UK Parliament, 2008).

Household income is another widely used measure of socio-economic position. Because different types of household need different levels of income to achieve the same standard of living, incomes are adjusted ('equivalized') to take account of the size and composition of the household. Income data can be used divide the population into income tertiles (thirds), as in Figure 2, and quintiles (fifths) as in Figure 1.

Area-based measures take information from individuals (like employment status) and households (like household income) and aggregate them at area level. The spatial unit can range from a small area, like a neighbourhood, through larger units, like countries, to global regions. Information across a variety of measures can be combined to form a composite indicator of area affluence and deprivation. One example is England's Indices of Multiple Deprivation (IMD) which combine indicators across domains, including income, employment, housing and health, into a single deprivation score (DCLG, 2008). England's health inequalities target for life expectancy (set for achievement by 2010) uses the IMD to identify disadvantaged areas. The IMD is used alongside an additional set of measures of health (male and female life expectancy alongside premature mortality from cancer and cardiovascular disease) to identify the 20 per cent of areas with the worst deprivation and health profile (DH, 2008).

As with other measures, area-based measures have their limitations. First, areas are socially mixed. Within poor areas, there are richer people, while rich areas are also home to poorer people. Further, residential patterns tend to vary across ethnic groups. In the UK, levels of residential concentration are lower among white groups than among Caribbeans and Indians, and are at their highest among Pakistanis (Robinson and Reeve, 2006). As noted in Chapter 1.4, the pattern of ethnic segregation is stronger still in the USA. Second, people's perceptions of their neighbourhood do not necessarily square with the official ratings. Residents may rate their neighbourhoods highly on dimensions that official deprivation indices fail to capture. One such dimension is feeling you belong. Feeling you belong can be particularly important for groups who experience stigma and discrimination in the wider society: even if unemployment rates are high and housing is poor, the local area can confer important psycho-social benefits (Pickett and Wilkinson, 2008).

Third, area-based measures mean that socio-economic factors relating to people's individual and household circumstances cannot be separated from factors operating at the area level. As Chapter 1.4 explains, health in poorer areas may be poorer simply because poorer people in poorer health are more likely to live there. Or the spatial patterning of health may reflect an additional toll that living in a poor area takes on people's health. The broad consensus is that individual and household socio-economic circumstances are the more powerful predictors of health but that areas have a small additional effect (Pickett and Pearl, 2001). This suggests that area-based measures of health inequalities will be capturing the influence of factors operating at multiple levels, including individual, household and neighbourhood (see Chapter 1.4).

Health inequalities: patterns and trends

Socio-economic inequalities are evident across space. Thus there are global health inequalities, with a 20-year difference in life expectancy between the 60 per cent of the world's population living in low-income countries and the one-sixth living in high-income countries (UNDP, 2007). There are health inequalities between countries: life expectancy is lower in the USA than the UK, and the UK's health record is poorer than Nordic countries like Sweden (UNDP, 2007). Health inequalities are found, too, within countries as Figures 1 and 2 illustrate.

Socio-economic inequalities also persist over time and across changes in the major causes of death. For example in 19th-century Britain, it was infectious diseases which underlay the social gradient in health, diseases linked to poor sanitation and overcrowding. From the late 19th century, the death-toll from infectious diseases fell rapidly, while deaths from the chronic diseases of later life, like circulatory disease (a category which combines coronary heart disease and stroke) and cancer, began to increase. In 1880, they were identified as the cause of 10 per cent of deaths in Britain. By 1900, the proportion had reached 25 per cent and peaked at over 70 per cent in the 1970s and 1980s. Today, over 60 per cent of deaths have cancer and circulatory disease as their underlying cause. Poor sanitation and overcrowding play little part in the development of these diseases; instead, a cluster of behaviours, including a high-fat, energy-dense diet, physical inactivity and cigarette smoking, are identified as the major risk factors (Lopez et al., 2006).

As the chronic disease epidemic took hold, its social profile changed. In the early 20th century, the limited evidence for the UK suggests that mortality rates from cancer and circulatory disease were either similar across socio-economic groups (lung cancer) or were higher in higher socio-economic groups (coronary heart disease) (Townsend and Davidson, 1982; Davey Smith, 1997). As the century progressed and death rates from chronic disease rose, the familiar social gradient started to emerge. By the 1960s, it was becoming evident among men for lung cancer mortality. Figure 4 picks up the story from the 1970s for coronary heart disease, the UK's leading cause of death. As it suggests, the social gradient has steepened over time because death rates have fallen much more rapidly in higher than lower socio-economic groups.

With inequalities in the major causes of death widening over time, it is not surprising that inequalities in overall mortality and life expectancy have also widened. Figure 5 points to the upward trend in life expectancy for men and women across the socio-economic spectrum. However, the

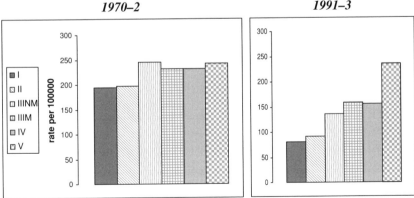

Figure 4 European standardized mortality rates by social class, men aged 20–64, coronary heart disease, England and Wales.
Source: Drever and Bunting (1997), Table 8.6.

Men: social class I, social class V and all men

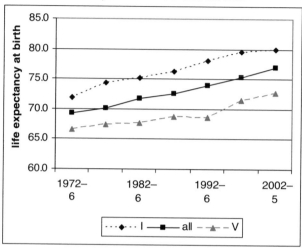

Women: social class I, social class V and all women

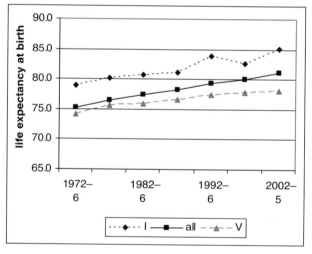

Figure 5 Life expectancy at birth, 1972–2005, England and Wales.
Source: ONS (2007), Table 1.

improvement in life expectancy has been more rapid among those at the top than the bottom of the socio-economic hierarchy. A similar pattern is evident in other high-income countries: more rapid declines in death rates in more advantaged socio-economic groups are widening socio-economic inequalities in mortality and life expectancy (Mackenbach, 2005).

Understanding health inequalities

How can the enduring association between socio-economic position and health be understood?

One possibility is that the association is a statistical artefact: an illusion resulting from flaws in the measurement of people's socio-economic position and in the statistical techniques through which its health effects are estimated. While measurement is never perfect, it is now widely accepted that statistical inaccuracies are insufficient to account for either the persistence or the magnitude of the social gradient.

Researchers have been mindful, too, that an individual's health influences, as well as is influenced by, their socio-economic circumstances. The onset of illness and impairment can force individuals into lower-paid work or out of the labour market, with their poorer circumstances placing their health further at risk – a process explored in Chapter 3.1. When downward social mobility occurs, it is likely to increase the rates of morbidity and mortality in lower socio-economic groups. Conversely, those in better health are more likely to move up the occupational ladder, amplifying the health advantages associated with higher socio-economic status. Health-related social mobility (or 'health selection' as it is also called) is estimated to make a small contribution to the overall socio-economic gradient in health (Power et al., 1996). However, it leaves the major part still to be explained.

The weight of evidence suggests that this major part reflects the influence of people's socio-economic circumstances on their health. Summarizing this evidence, Bruce Link and Jo Phelan (1995) concluded that social position is a 'fundamental cause' of health. The distinguishing feature of such a cause is its persisting association with health across time and place, and despite changes in the major causes of death. Fundamental causes 'affect multiple disease outcomes through multiple mechanisms, and consequently maintain an association with disease even when intervening mechanisms change' (1995: 80). In other words, diseases can change (infectious diseases can give way to chronic diseases) and mechanisms can change (for example, from environmental threats like poor sanitation to behavioural factors like sedentary lifestyles and cigarette smoking) but the association with socio-economic position endures.

Noting that the association persists is not, of course, the same thing as explaining how it persists. While perspectives vary in detail, the broad consensus is that the social gradient in health endures because, although societies and causes of death change over time, an individual's socio-economic position still determines their access to resources which promote health and their exposure to risks which damage it. As a result, socio-economic advantage continues to bring more by way of health-enhancing resources and less by way of health-damaging exposures; in contrast, socio-economic disadvantage restricts access to the resources which promote health and leaves the individual more exposed to health risks (Power and Matthews, 1997).

This clustering of risks means that children growing up in poor circumstances are more likely to have other experiences which also damage their health (see Chapters 1.1 and 1.2). A British study following families over a 4-year period from 2000 to 2004 provides an example. It identified a group of children in persistent poverty, defined as living in a household with an income below the official poverty line (of 60% of equivalized household income before housing costs) in at least three of the four years. Twelve per cent of families met this criterion, a group of children who were additionally vulnerable to a range of other adverse experiences (Barnes et al., 2008). For example, they were much more likely to live in 'bad housing' (defined as living in temporary accommodation currently or in the past year, living in over-crowded accommodation and/or living in unfit accommodation), to have less than an hour of physical activity a week, and to be at increased risk of social exclusion, as measured by school expulsion or suspension in the previous 12 months.

In adulthood, too, those with limited economic resources are most exposed to health-related risks. Compared with the highest NS-SEC group (people in managerial and professional occupations), those in routine and manual work have lower earnings, less stable earnings, and poorer working conditions (Goldthorpe and McKnight, 2006). They are at much greater risk of unemployment and, particularly, of recurrent and long-term unemployment (Goldthorpe and McKnight, 2006), an experience which is also know to be detrimental to health (Bartley and Owen, 1996). The clustering of risks does not end with ones related to the labour market. Socio-economic disadvantage is also associated with health risks at home, for example, with poor housing and exposure to air pollution (see Chapter 1.2). Behavioural risks follow the same pattern: those who enjoy better working and living conditions are less likely to smoke and to have a poor diet and a sedentary lifestyle. The socio-economic gradient in cigarette smoking is discussed in Chapters 2.3 and 3.2; Figure 6 therefore focuses on diet and physical activity. A healthy diet is measured by the consumption of the UK government's recommendation of five portions of fruit and vegetables a day, and low physical activity by taking 30 minutes of moderate or vigorous activity – which can include housework, manual work, sports and exercise, gardening and DIY, and walking – less than once a week on average.

Health-damaging factors not only cluster, they also accumulate over time (see Chapters 1.1 and 1.2). For example, the powerful influence of family background on children's future socio-economic position means

Five or more portions of fruit and vegetables per day

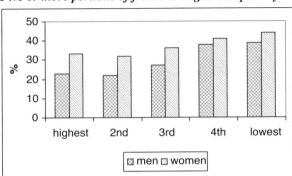

Low physical activity

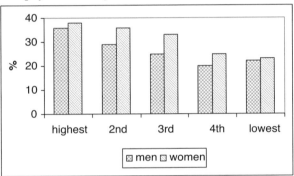

Figure 6 Daily fruit and vegetable consumption (≥ 5 portions) and low physical activity (≤ 30 minutes per week) among adults aged 16 and over by equivalized household income, England, 2006.
Source: Craig and Mindell (2008), Tables 6.3 and 7.3.

that children born into poorer circumstances are more likely to experience social disadvantage across their lives than those born into more advantaged circumstances. These generational continuities in disadvantage are found across high-income societies but are more evident in some countries, like the UK and the USA, than in others, like the Nordic countries (Graham, 2007). Inequalities in young people's educational trajectories, and in their educational attainment in particular, are known to play an important role in these continuities. In other words, social background influences social prospects indirectly, with an advantaged start in life helping children gain the educational qualifications they need to access jobs in the higher echelons of the labour market. In the poorest 20 per cent of families in Britain, less than 10 per cent of young people have a degree by the age of 23; among the richest 20 per cent, the proportion is over 40 per cent (Blanden and Machin, 2007).

While much of the focus has been on education, it is not the only route through which advantage and disadvantage is transmitted across the generations. Young people's domestic pathways are also important, and are particularly important for women. Being and remaining married matters more for women's living standards than for men's, and exit from marriage brings a greater and more rapid fall in income. Becoming a parent has a greater impact on women's employment and earnings, and women are also more likely to become a lone parent and devote a larger part of their lives to caring for children alone (Graham, 2007). In recent decades, women's domestic pathways have become much more varied; they are also increasingly patterned by their social background, a trend evident across high-income countries. For example, as discussed in Chapter 2.4, longer years of education have meant that young women and men from advantaged backgrounds are delaying both marriage and having children, while young people growing up in poorer circumstances are more likely to become parents by their mid-twenties and outside marriage (Singh et al., 2001).

Drawn from a contemporary British study of women, Figure 7 illustrates how childhood circumstances influence both women's educational and domestic pathways into adulthood. It focuses on women aged 22 to 34 and uses the NS-SEC as the measure of their childhood circumstances (based on father's occupation when the survey participants were children). While only a minority of women had no educational qualifications and was a mother before the age of 22, it points to marked socio-economic gradients in women's educational and domestic trajectories.

Two points are worth noting about the evidence on social and health inequalities reviewed in this introductory chapter. First, a higher risk of an outcome in poorer groups – of becoming a young mother, for example – does not mean that it will inevitably occur. As Figure 7 indicates, the experience may only happen to a minority, even among those in the poorest circumstances. What a higher risk suggests, however, is that the outcome is more common among children and adults in disadvantaged circumstances than among those in more advantaged circumstances and among the population as a whole. Second, quantitative data reveal little about people's everyday lives. Researchers have therefore turned to qualitative studies to understand the choices and constraints that underlie the associations between social disadvantage and individual behaviours. For example, Chapter 2.3 discusses the insights that can be gleaned from qualitative studies of cigarette smoking while Chapter 2.4 explores how

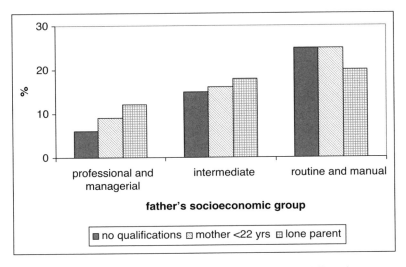

Figure 7 Educational and domestic trajectories by childhood socio-economic circumstances (based on father's occupation), women aged 22 to 34, Britain 1998–2002.
Notes: 1. Childhood socio-economic circumstances based on father's occupation at the time of the woman's birth, categorized using NS-SEC.
2. Percentage of lone parents based is based on women who were mothers at time of recruitment to survey.
Source: unpublished data reproduced with permission of Southampton Women's Survey.

young women from different social backgrounds negotiate sexual and re-productive behaviour.

An overview of the chapters

The book tackles the task of understanding health inequalities in three sections. Part 1 reviews evidence on health inequalities over time and place. Chapters 1.1 and 1.2 draw on what is a called a 'life-course perspective', a perspective which sheds light on how inequalities in people's circumstances influence their health from the early years of life, across adulthood and into older age. Catherine Law discusses how a life-course perspective underlines the importance of childhood for children's current and future well-being. She presents evidence of socio-economic and ethnic inequalities in the determinants of health at this crucial life stage and notes the potential for government policies to promote child health to have unintended negative consequences. Mel Bartley and David Blane take a life-course approach to health and health inequalities in older age. They outline the social and biological processes through which people's health can be influenced by social circumstances across their lives, pointing to the long-term effects of earlier circumstances on physical health in later life.

Chapters 1.3 and 1.4 are concerned with socio-economic inequalities in health captured at area level. Danny Dorling and Bethan Thomas's chapter provides new analyses of geographical inequalities in mortality in Britain from 1921. They note the marked widening of geographical inequalities in health through the 1980s and 1990s, with high levels of inequalities continuing up to 2004–6, and consider the implications for policy. Continuing the focus on place, Sally Macintyre and Anne Ellaway consider the different ways in which neighbourhoods may influence people and their health. Reviewing research on one key health resource – access to fresh and nutritious food – they point the way to a deeper understanding of area influences.

Link and Phelan's (1995) 'fundamental causes of health' are not restricted to socio-economic position. They encompass all social positions which embody unequal access to societal resources and unequal exposure to health risks. Ethnicity and gender therefore qualify as fundamental causes of people's (unequal) health. Part 2 of the book focuses on these inequalities.

Chapters 2.1 and 2.2 address the intersections between socio-economic position and religious and ethnic identities. James Nazroo and Saffron Karlsen highlight both inequalities in health between religious groups and ethnic inequalities within religious groups. Their analyses suggest that the socio-economic disadvantages faced by some religious/ethnic minorities contribute to these health inequalities, with experiences of racism, and perceptions of living in a racist society also related to health outcomes for religious minority groups. Karl Atkin continues the exploration of the intersections around ethnic and religious identities in his chapter, this time through qualitative research. He draws on two studies involving participants from minority groups, the first exploring how young people with hearing impairments negotiate and celebrate their cultural and ethnic identities and the second exploring how religion and faith influence decisions about antenatal screening for sickle cell and thalassaemia disorders.

Chapters 2.3 and 2.4 turn the spotlight on how gender and socio-economic inequality influence people's lives and people's health. Kate Hunt and David Batty present a new review of socio-economic inequalities in mortality among men and women as well as analyses of the gendered socio-economic patterning of two health behaviours, cigarette smoking and binge drinking. They note how these behaviours are expressive of gendered class identities, and how their cultural meanings have changed over time. Naomi Rudoe and Rachel Thomson continue the exploration of the cultural meanings of behaviours lying at the intersections between gender and socio-economic inequalities, this time through qualitative studies involving young people. They focus on a behaviour which is widely regarded as 'the wrong thing to do'. They explore the meanings of becoming a teenage parent for young people and for young women who become mothers. In so doing, the chapter underlines the importance of understanding individual behaviour within the context of people's everyday lives.

Policy implications are discussed through Part 1 and Part 2, and are explicitly addressed in Part 3. Margaret Whitehead and colleagues take the example of how policies can impact unequally on people who have long-term illnesses and disabilities. Discussing how ill health and impairment can have more damaging consequences for the employment opportunities and socio-economic circumstances of those who are already disadvantaged, they consider the role of different types of policy in magnifying or preventing such adverse consequences. Hilary Graham's introductory chapter focuses on living standards and cigarette smoking, and considers evidence of how policies can moderate (or increase) socio-economic inequalities in these two key determinants of health. Common themes emerge from the analysis, suggesting that policies have a major influence on the social distribution of health determinants.

Taken together, the chapters provide powerful evidence that social inequalities are embodied in individual health: in our physical functioning, psycho-social well-being and vulnerability to disease and disability. While these embodied inequalities are found in all societies, it is clear that their scale varies over time and between countries. As this suggests, health inequalities are not immutable: policies can and do make a difference.

References

Barnes, M., Conolly, A. and Tomaszewski, W. (2008) *The Circumstances of Persistently Poor Families with Children,* Research Report No 487. London: Department for Work and Pensions.

Bartley, M. and Owen, C. (1996) Relation between socio-economic status, employment and health during economic change 1973–93, *British Medical Journal*, 313: 445–9.

Blanden, J. and Machin, S. (2007) *Recent Changes in Intergenerational Mobility in Britain*. London: Sutton Trust.

Craig, R. and Mindell, J. (eds) (2008) *Health Survey for England 2006 Volume 1: Cardiovascular Disease and Risk Factors in Adults*. London: National Centre for Social Research.

Davey Smith, G. (1997) Socio-economic differentials, in D.L. Kuh and Y. Ben-Shlomo (eds) *A Life Course Approach to Chronic Disease Epidemiology*. Oxford: Oxford University Press.

Department for Communities and Local Government (DCLG) (2008) *The English Indices of Deprivation 2007*. London: DCLG.

Department of Health (DH) (2008) *Tackling Health Inequalities: 2007 Status Report on the Programme for Action*. London: DH.

Douglas, J.W.B. and Blomfield, J.M. (1958) *Children Under Five*. London: George Allen and Unwin.

Drever, F. and Bunting, J. (1997) Patterns and trends in male mortality, in F. Drever and M. Whitehead (eds) *Health Inequalities*. London: Office for National Statistics.

Goldthorpe, J.H. and McKnight, A. (2006) The economic basis of social class, in S.L. Morgan, D.B. Grusky and G.S. Fields (eds) *Mobility and Inequality*. Stanford, CA: Stanford University Press.

Graham, H. (2007) *Unequal Lives: Health and Socioeconomic Inequalities*. Maidenhead: Open University Press.

Lancet (1843) Editorial, *The Lancet*, 1040: 657–61.

Link, B.G. and Phelan, J. (1995) Social conditions as fundamental causes of disease, *Journal of Health and Social Behaviour*, extra issue: 80–94.

Lopez, A.D., Mathers, C.D., Ezzati, M., Jamison, D.T. and Murray, C.J.L. (2006) *Global Burden of Disease and Risk Factors*. Oxford: Oxford University Press and World Bank.

Lopez, A.D., Salomon, J., Ahmad, O., Murray, C.J.L. and Mafat, D. (2001) *Life Tables for 191 Countries: Data, Methods and Results*, discussion paper no 9. Geneva: World Health Organization.

Mackenbach, J.P. (2005) *Health Inequalities: Europe in Profile*. Rotterdam: Erasmus MC University Medical Center.

Machin, S. (2003) Unto them that hath . . . , *CentrePiece*, 8(1): 5–9.

Office for National Statistics (ONS) (2007) *Trends in ONS Longitudinal Study Estimates of Life Expectancy by Social Class*. London: The Stationery Office.

Organization for Economic Co-operation and Development (OECD) (2008) *Growing Unequal? Income Distribution and Poverty in OECD Countries*. Paris: OECD.

Pickett, K.E. and Pearl, M. (2001) Multilevel analyses of neighbourhood socioeconomic context and health outcomes: critical review, *Journal of Epidemiology and Community Health*, 55: 111–22.

Pickett, K.E. and Wilkinson, R.G (2008) People like us: ethnic group density effects on health, *Ethnicity and Health*, 13(4): 321–34.

Pollitt, R.A., Rose, K.M. and Kaufman, J.S. (2005) Evaluating the evidence for models of life course socio-economic factors and cardiovascular outcomes: a systematic review, *BMC Public Health*, 5(7): 1–13.

Power, C., Matthews, S. and Manor, O. (1996) Inequalities in self-rated health in the 1958 birth cohort: lifetime social circumstances or social mobility? *British Medical Journal*, 313: 449–53.

Power, C. and Matthews, S. (1997) Origins of health inequalities in a national population sample, *Lancet*, 350: 1584–9.

Robinson, D. and Reeve, K. (2006) *Neighbourhood Experiences of New Immigration.* Sheffield: Centre for Regional Economic and Social Research, Sheffield Hallam University.

Rose, D. and Pevalin, D.J. (eds) (2003) *A Researcher's Guide to The National Statistics Socio-economic Classification.* London: SAGE.

Royal Commission on the Health of Towns (1845) *First Report of Commissioners of Inquiry into the State of Large Towns and Populous Districts.* London: Royal Commission on the Health of Towns.

Singh, S., Darroch, J.E., Frost, J.J. and the Study Team (2001) Socioeconomic disadvantage and adolescent women's sexual and reproductive behaviour: the case of five developed countries, *Family Planning Perspectives*, 33(6): 251–8.

Sproston, K. and Mindell, J. (eds) (2006) *Health Survey for England 2004: The Health of Minority Ethnic Groups.* Leeds: The Information Centre.

Sproston, K. and Primatesta, P. (2004) *Health Survey for England 2003, Volume 2: Risk Factors for Cardiovascular Disease.* London: Office for National Statistics.

Townsend, P. and Davidson, P. (eds) (1982) *Inequalities in Health: The Black Report.* Harmondsworth: Penguin.

UK Parliament (2008) *Human Fertilisation and Embryology Bill [HL] 2007–2008, as Amended in the Committee and in Public Committee.* Available at: www.publications.parliament.uk/pa/cm200708/cmbills/120/08120.i-iv.html.

United Nations Development Programme (UNDP) (2007) *Human Development Report 2007/2008.* New York: UNDP.

Part 1

Health inequalities: understanding patterns over time and place

The chapters in Part 1 of the book underline the importance of time and place for understanding health inequalities.

Two chapters – by Catherine Law and by Mel Bartley and David Blane – are centrally concerned with time. They discuss how an appreciation of time, and of individual lifetimes in particular, is contributing to explanations of health inequalities. They do so by introducing the concept of life-course. The concept draws attention to how people's health is shaped by the course of their lives, with life-course research illuminating the processes through which social inequalities in infancy, adulthood and older age all have their part to play in the socio-economic gradient in health.

An appreciation of time is particularly important in societies where chronic diseases, like heart disease and cancer, are the major killers. These are diseases with complex aetiologies where multiple factors are often involved and where there can be time-lags of years or even decades between exposure and evidence of effect. An appreciation of life course and biography is also needed to inform the development of policy. If the life course matters – for example, if disadvantage in early life has life-long effects on life chances and health chances – then policies which tackle inequalities in people's circumstances across their lives are an essential part of an equity-oriented public health strategy.

Two chapters – by Danny Dorling and Bethan Thomas and by Sally Macintyre and Anne Ellaway – are centrally concerned with place and, particularly, the places in which people live. Their chapters are set against a backcloth of the spatial polarization of poverty and affluence in the UK, on the one hand, and government investment in area-based strategies to tackle social and health inequalities, on the other.

The chapter by Danny Dorling and Bethan Thomas combines a focus on place with a consideration of trends in area inequalities over time. It reviews evidence on geographical inequalities in health in Britain across the last hundred years. The chapter by Sally Macintyre and Anne Ellaway outlines the processes through which areas can influence the health of those that live there, illustrating the processes through a focus on access to a key health resource, namely nutritious food.

1.1 Life-course influences on children's futures

Catherine Law

Introduction

> *The true measure of a nation's standing is how well it attends to its children – their health and safety, their material security, their education and socialization, and their sense of being loved, valued, and included in the families and societies in which they are born.*

So opens UNICEF's report card on child well-being in rich countries (UNICEF Innocenti Research Centre, 2007). The report goes on to describe huge variations between countries in the well-being of their child populations, with the USA and UK consistently in the lowest-ranked countries for most domains. In a further analysis of the UNICEF data, Pickett and Wilkinson (2007) note that the overall index of well-being, and several of its domains, including health, are related not to mean income but to income inequality, with poorer levels of health and well-being in rich countries with more unequal incomes. It is a paradox that the increasing wealth of nations has not necessarily been accompanied by overall improvements in children's health and that within some, if not all, rich nations, the health and other benefits of national prosperity are not shared equally (Li et al., 2008). For example, in the UK the prevalence of mental health problems is increasing and their distribution is socially patterned. Mental health problems are more common in children living in families with a low educational or occupational status (British Medical Association, 2006).

However, to appreciate the true impact of inequality on the health of individuals, it is necessary to consider the whole of their lives. A life-course approach, which has its origins in the discipline of epidemiology, does this. Life-course epidemiology is the study of long-term biological, behavioural and psycho-social processes that link adult health and disease risk to physical or social exposures acting during gestation, childhood, adolescence, earlier in adult life, or across generations (Kuh and

Ben-Shlomo, 1997). Although life-course epidemiology has traditionally focused on health in later adult life, there is no reason not to apply such an approach to earlier periods of individuals' lives, and in relation to both their current and future health. For example, consider the current rising prevalence of childhood obesity. As well as its immediate impacts on children's health and well-being (Lobstein et al., 2004), childhood obesity predicts adult obesity (Parsons et al., 1999). If current trends in obesity are maintained, it is estimated that the development of type 2 diabetes in about one-third of today's birth cohort in the USA will significantly shorten life expectancy and increase morbidity (Olshansky et al., 2005). Given that childhood obesity is socially patterned (Shrewsbury and Wardle, 2008), this reduction in life expectancy may be expected to exacerbate current differences in longevity between social groups.

A life-course approach also recognizes the unusually high number of critical or sensitive periods during childhood and adolescence. A critical period occurs when there are rapid and usually irreversible changes towards greater complexity taking place. Influences in these periods can have long-lasting, permanent effects. A sensitive period is also a period of rapid change, but one in which there is some scope to modify, or even reverse, the changes at a later time (Kuh and Ben-Shlomo, 1997). Fetuses, infants, children, and adolescents pass through many critical and sensitive periods as they develop to maturity, particularly between conception and early childhood. This makes not only pregnancy but also childhood and adolescence, particularly in the early years, an unparalleled time during which external influences, both good and bad, can influence an individual's health and well-being across their whole life. Of particular importance is the health and circumstances of mothers, which links to their children's health through biological, behavioural and social mechanisms (Kuh and Ben-Shlomo, 1997).

A life-course approach illuminates the role of childhood disadvantage in determining adult health and inequalities in adult health. Graham and Power (2004) describe two main pathways through which childhood disadvantage results in poor adult health. First, childhood circumstances may influence adult circumstances which in turn affect adult health. For example, poor educational attainment is associated with increased risk of unemployment, and joblessness is associated with poor adult health. Second, the circumstances that children experience as they grow up influence their childhood health and development (considered in their widest sense, to include mental, social and emotional health as well as physical health and health behaviours). Good childhood health tends to lead to good adult health and vice versa. For example, a mother living in disadvantaged circumstances has a high risk of giving birth to a low birth weight child, and

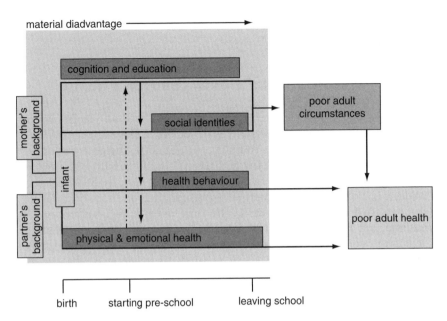

material diadvantage

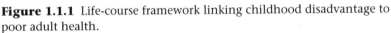

birth   starting pre-school   leaving school

Figure 1.1.1 Life-course framework linking childhood disadvantage to poor adult health.
Source: Graham and Power (2004: figure 7), reproduced with permission from the publishers.

low birth weight is associated with a range of adverse health outcomes in childhood as well as adult life (Graham and Power, 2004). Graham and Power describe how earlier or current disadvantage shapes interlinked trajectories through childhood, during which resources are accumulated or lost, and development is optimized or harmed (Figure 1.1.1). The trajectories describe pathways related to physical and emotional health, health behaviours, social identities, and cognition and education.

The chapter will first consider how inequalities in the determinants of health are affecting children's health and life chances now. It will focus on indicators which illustrate the extent to which variability in the trajectories of childhood experience conceptualized by Graham and Power (Figure 1.1.1) is relevant today. While the data presented relate mainly to England and to younger children, many of the patterns are found throughout the UK and in other rich countries like the USA as well as in older children and adolescents. The chapter will then present examples of analyses from the Millennium Cohort Study which demonstrate that inequalities in the life chances of children of the new century still exist, despite government commitments to eradicate them, and how policies and practice may address these.

Socio-economic inequalities in children's health

Infant mortality is inversely related to living standards and so has been a useful indicator of how circumstances in society at large affect children's health (Ferguson et al., 2006). To reflect this, in 2001, the government set a target for England to reduce inequalities in infant mortality, by narrowing the gap in infant mortality by at least 10 per cent by 2010 between children in the routine and manual group (defined as those with fathers who recorded their occupations at the time of birth registration as routine/manual) and the population as a whole. However, despite this policy focus and overall falls in infant mortality for all social groups since the baseline year for the target (1997–9), inequalities in infant mortality have increased over the last ten years. The infant mortality rate among routine and manual groups was 17 per cent higher than in the total population in 2004–6 compared to 13 per cent higher in 1997–9 (DH, 2008). A widening of the gap in infant mortality between socio-economic groups has also been observed in the USA. For the period 1985–9, infants in the most 'deprived' group (defined according to indicators representing local educational, occupational, economic and housing conditions) had a 36 per cent higher risk of neonatal mortality than infants in the least deprived group, which increased to a 46 per cent higher relative risk during 1995–2000 (Singh and Kogan, 2007).

Other indicators of early health in UK children also show persisting inequalities. For example, poorer mothers are more likely to give birth to smaller babies or to deliver before term (Spencer, 2003). Cerebral palsy, the most common childhood physical disability, occurs at higher rates in families with lower socio-economic position (Dolk et al., 2001), as does both unintentional (Ferguson et al., 2006) and non-accidental injury (Cawson et al., 2000), and emotional and behavioural problems (Meltzer et al., 2000). Childhood obesity, sometimes described as one of the greatest threats to public health, is also more common among disadvantaged children (Shrewsbury and Wardle, 2008).

Socio-economic inequalities in children's health behaviours

Compared to later adult life, childhood after infancy is a period of relatively low mortality and morbidity. However, childhood is also a time when health behaviours become established and so inequalities in health behaviours of children or their families are particularly important. Even in early childhood, socio-economic patterns are emerging.

Overall, there is reasonable evidence that children from poorer families are eating a less healthy diet than their richer peers (Batty and Leon, 2002). For example, young children from families in poorer socio-economic circumstances are less likely to eat the recommended amount of fruit and vegetables and more likely to eat burgers, chips and sugary confectionery than children from more advantaged families (Nessa and Gallagher, 2004). However, patterns in physical activity are less clear. There is some evidence that sedentary behaviour is more common in children, particularly girls, from less well-off families (see, for example, Brodersen et al., 2007) but inconsistent findings in relation to physical activity (Batty and Leon, 2002; Ferguson et al., 2006). The social patterning of sedentary behaviour is of particular concern when set against the backdrop of the high overall levels of sedentary leisure activity reported by children now.

Parents are a critical influence in establishing health behaviours. For example, children are much more likely to smoke if one or both parents are a smoker (Fuller, 2007). Similarly, the presence of parental obesity is a strong predictor of childhood obesity which persists into adulthood (Lake et al., 1997). While shared genes may play a role, environmental factors relating to diet and physical activity are also influential, and are critical in the expression of some genetic tendencies to being overweight (Lobstein et al., 2004). Both smoking and obesity in adulthood (particularly in women) are socially patterned, with higher rates in disadvantaged groups (Craig and Mindell, 2008). Thus the strong relationships in smoking and obesity within families leads to inter-generational transmission of inequalities in health disorders which are associated with cigarette smoking and overweight, particularly as smoking in pregnancy is also a risk factor for offspring obesity. A further parental behavioural influence on young children's health is infant feeding. Mothers from lower socio-economic groups are less likely to start or continue breastfeeding, and they also tend to introduce solid foods earlier than mothers from more advantaged families (Griffiths et al., 2005; Ferguson et al., 2006; Bolling et al., 2007). Similar patterns are found in the USA. In the 2005/06 birth cohort of the US National Health and Nutrition Examination Survey, 57 per cent of infants from families of lower income had been 'ever breastfed' compared with 74 per cent of infants from higher income families. Breastfeeding was also significantly more likely among Mexican American (80%) and non-Hispanic white (79%) infants compared with non-Hispanic black infants (65%) (McDowell et al., 2008).

Inequalities in the determinants of health in childhood

The data presented so far show that socio-economic differences in health status and health behaviours in childhood are widespread. If all of the population, including children, occupied similar socio-economic positions then these differences would have a small impact on public health. Unfortunately, this is not the case. This section will demonstrate that there are marked discrepancies in the material circumstances of children's lives which are likely to have profound influences on their health.

The last ten years has seen unprecedented commitment to tackle child poverty in the UK, with the aim of eliminating it by 2020 (DWP, 2006). This commitment is supported by all the major political parties. While there has been progress, what is striking is the number of children still living in poverty. In 2006–7, 2.9 million children were living in poverty using the government's measure (household income below 60% median income before housing costs) (Brewer et al., 2008). Although this is 500,000 fewer than in 1996–7, it remains an unacceptably high figure. Children remain disproportionately represented in low-income households in the UK and some children are particularly at risk of experiencing poverty. These include children in lone-parent families, in families where the parents work less than full-time or are unemployed, those in families of more than two children, and those whose mother is under 25 years old (DWP, 2007). Many children in the USA also live in poverty. Eighteen per cent (13.2 million) of all children in the USA in 2007 were classified as living below the 'federal poverty level' (US $21,200 for a family of four, US $17,600 for a family of three, or US $14,000 for a family of two), with a further 21 per cent (15.6 million) in families whose income was less than twice the federal poverty level (Douglas-Hall and Chau, 2008).

The poor material circumstances in which many children live their lives are documented in the quality of their homes. Twenty-eight per cent of social tenants and almost a third of vulnerable private households (those receiving one of the main means-tested or disability-related benefits) live in dwellings which do not meet standards required to be classified as a 'decent' home (DCLG, 2008), with children disproportionately represented within these households. Furthermore, the number of homeless families with children living in temporary accommodation remains fairly constant (around 60,000) although great improvements have been made in reducing the number of families having to live in bed and breakfast accommodation (DH, 2008).

Differentials in educational achievement have been identified as one of the main determinants of inequalities in health (WHO, 2008) and tackling educational inequalities is one of the most politically acceptable policy solutions in the UK. There is some evidence that investment in education focused on disadvantaged areas may be closing the gap in educational achievement. For example, the proportion of pupils achieving good GCSE passes (equivalent to five GCSE grades at A* to C) has increased for all children over the last five years, from 49 per cent in 2002 to 59 per cent in 2007. The increase among children who are eligible for free school meals (a means-tested benefit) has been more marked – from 23 per cent in 2002 to 35 per cent in 2007. However, there is still a large difference in achievement between children from disadvantaged families and their better-off peers. The picture for looked-after children in England is even bleaker, with their rate of good passes at GCSE being less than 13 per cent (DCSF, 2008).

Children's health also varies according to where they live. Place differences are particularly important in developing policy to tackle health inequalities because area-level differences are often easier to measure and monitor than individual differences. Furthermore, policies can be targeted at areas through existing delivery mechanisms and settings (for example, through financial allocations to local authorities and directives to schools) rather than at individuals. As an example of variability in child health at regional level, in 2002–4, overall mortality rates for children and young people up to 19 years of age ranged from 41 per 100,000 in the South East of England to 58.6 per 100,000 in the West Midlands. Other child health indicators showed marked regional variations but not necessarily in the same directions. For instance, the West Midlands had the lowest mean number of missing decayed or filled teeth in five-year-old children (1.02) and the North West the highest (2.17). In contrast, London had the highest under-18 years conception rate and the East of England the lowest (Ferguson et al., 2006).

Place differences reflect a complex mix of differences in geography, quality of the environment, and characteristics of the people who live there (see Chapters 1.3 and 1.4). This is well illustrated by a recent analysis of infant mortality and its risk factors across London primary care trusts (PCTs). There were marked variations between PCTs in rates of infant deaths and also in risk factors for infant deaths such as area-level deprivation, breastfeeding, and smoking in pregnancy, but these were not always coincident. For example, Haringey had the highest infant mortality of any London PCT in 2003–5 and relatively high rates of smoking in pregnancy. However, it also had high rates of breastfeeding, a protective factor for infant mortality. Eighty-six per cent of Haringey mothers started to breastfeed their babies compared to a range for all London PCTs of 51–91 per cent (London Health Observatory, 2007). The apparent mismatch between area-level infant mortality and some of its risk factors is probably due to the ethnic mix of residents. Haringey has a high proportion of mothers from minority ethnic groups as well as having many areas of disadvantage within its boundaries. Infants from minority ethnic groups are likely to be breastfed, but are also at high risk of low birth weight and congenital anomalies, risk factors for infant mortality which are not influenced by breastfeeding.

Looking back at Figure 1.1.1, it is apparent that the data presented so far in this chapter do not indicate an optimistic future for many UK children or for the health of the nation. Many children are experiencing the adverse health, education, social and behavioural trajectories that accompany disadvantage and that will, if unchecked, lead to poor adult health. Yet with each new birth comes the opportunity for change. The remainder of the chapter will focus on analyses of children of the new century, members of the Millennium Cohort Study (MCS). Through specific examples, it will illustrate how inequalities in health are persisting and how analysis of cohorts such as the MCS can inform policies to address them.

An introduction to the Millennium Cohort Study

The Millennium Cohort Study (MCS) is the most recent in a valuable series of UK cohort studies (Centre for Longitudinal Studies, 2008). It aims to study the influence of society on children's lives now and into the future and there are aspirations to follow the cohort for decades. Unlike the birth cohort studies of 1946, 1958, and 1970, the Millennium Cohort focuses on a cohort of children identified at nine months of age, but for whom there is good recalled data of pregnancy and birth. A particular feature of MCS is the relatively high numbers of children from minority ethnic groups and from disadvantaged areas, both groups that have been under-represented in previous cohorts and in research more generally. Thus it presents one of the best opportunities so far to study inequalities in health using a life-course approach.

There were 18,819 children in the original cohort. So far data have been collected and made available from MCS children when they were nine months, three years (14,630 children), and five years (12,989). In addition, in 2007 and 2008 data were collected on the children at age seven years and will become available in due course. A wide range of data was and is being collected – for example, on the material and financial circumstances of families, characteristics of the areas where children live, how they get on at school and relate to their peers, the health of family members and so on. A great strength of the MCS is that, in the future, all of the trajectories – physical, social, educational and behavioural – postulated to influence adult health across the life course can be examined separately and together. The examples of analyses presented here will focus on physical health and health behaviours up to three years.

Inequalities in immunization

Immunization is a highly cost-effective health service intervention to protect individuals and promote public health. Such protection often lasts for life, and protects children from early diseases, some of which have long-term consequences. Childhood immunization rates are generally high in the UK, and over the last 50 years increasing numbers of safe and effective vaccines have been introduced. However, in 1998, a research study was published which was widely interpreted as showing a link between the measles, mumps and rubella vaccine (MMR), a vaccine recommended by the government for nearly all children, and both autism and bowel disease (Wakefield et al., 1998). Following this, levels of immunization with the MMR vaccine declined dramatically, although some parents opted for single vaccines against measles, mumps and rubella instead.

Before the 1998 'scare', immunization rates showed marked inequalities, with lower rates in lone-parent and larger families, and for children living in disadvantaged areas. After 1998, the inequalities in vaccine uptake were lessened. Unfortunately, this was because of declining rates of uptake among advantaged families, rather than increased uptake in disadvantaged families (Middleton and Baker, 2003). Paradoxically, this decline in inequalities in vaccine uptake increased the absolute risk of vaccine-preventable disease in disadvantaged children, because the level of vaccination in the population as a whole was not sufficient to ensure herd immunity (where sufficient numbers of the population are immunized to prevent pathogen transmission), making epidemics among unimmunized children more likely. The MCS was unusual in collecting not only information on MMR but also on single measles, mumps and rubella vaccines. These data were used to assess the geographic, socio-economic and cultural risk factors for not accepting MMR (Pearce et al., 2008).

In the cohort overall, 88.6 per cent of children had been immunized with MMR by age three years, 5.2 per cent had received at least one of the single vaccines, and 6.1 per cent were unimmunized. Regression models were used to compare children who had received MMR with those who were completely unimmunized and also to compare those who had received MMR with those who had received one or more single vaccines. Table 1.1.1 shows some of the variables that predicted being unimmunized or receiving single vaccines, compared to being immunized with the recommended schedule of MMR vaccine.

Table 1.1.1 Adjusted risk ratios (RR)* and 95 per cent confidence intervals (CI) for immunization status

Social characteristics†	Column A			Column B		
	%‡ (No.)	Adjusted RR‡ (95% CI) for being unimmunized against MMR~	p-value	%‡ (No.)	Adjusted RR‡ (95% CI) for being immunized with at least one single antigen vaccine~	p-value
Maternal age at cohort birth						
14–19	8 (1101)	1.41 (1.08 to 1.85)		7 (1021)	0.14 (0.05 to 0.36)	
20–24	17 (2544)	1.07 (0.86 to 1.31)		17 (2431)	0.63 (0.45 to 0.87)	
25–29	28 (3874)	1		28 (3826)	1	
30–34	30 (4175)	1.11 (0.91 to 1.34)	<0.001	31 (4186)	1.36 (1.11 to 1.66)	<0.001
35–39	15 (1991)	1.60 (1.32 to 1.95)		15 (1933)	1.40 (1.10 to 1.77)	
≥40	2 (293)	2.34 (1.70 to 3.23)		2 (284)	3.04 (2.05 to 4.50)	
Single parent						
No	85 (11678)	1			Not related	
Yes	15 (2148)	1.31 (1.07 to 1.60)	<0.001			
Household income (£)						
<10400		Not related		22 (3068)	1	
10400–20800				32 (4118)	1.20 (0.86 to 1.69)	
20800–31200				22 (2639)	1.88 (1.33 to 2.66)	<0.001
31200–52000				17 (1974)	2.05 (1.42 to 2.95)	
≥52000				7 (694)	2.98 (2.05 to 4.32)	

Maternal education	Column A % (n)	Column A adjusted risk ratio	p	Column B % (n)	Column B adjusted risk ratio	p
None	16 (2477)	1		15 (2043)	1	
Other	2 (361)	1.06 (0.68 to 1.66)		2 (293)	1.76 (0.66 to 4.66)	
GCSE grades D–G	11 (1502)	0.81 (0.62 to 1.06)		11 (1343)	1.48 (0.74 to 2.97)	
O level/GCSE grades A*–C	35 (4664)	0.98 (0.81 to 1.19)	0.01	35 (4258)	2.66 (1.52 to 4.66)	<0.001
A/AS level	9 (1323)	1.35 (1.01 to 1.80)		10 (1230)	3.37 (1.85 to 6.13)	
Diploma	9 (1222)	1.15 (0.87 to 1.54)		10 (1161)	3.31 (1.92 to 5.69)	
Degree	17 (2277)	1.41 (1.05 to 1.89)		18 (2165)	3.15 (1.78 to 5.58)	
Ever smoked in pregnancy						
No	65 (9004)	1			Not related	
Yes	35 (4822)	1.22 (1.04 to 1.43)	0.02			

*An adjusted risk ratio shows the relative increase in risk associated with a factor, after adjusting for all effect of full other factors. For example in this table, children were 31% more likely not to be immunised if their mother was a lone parent compared to if their mother had a partner, after taking into account the other factors in the model such as age and income.

Notes

‡Percentages and risk ratios calculated with sample and non-response weights.

†Variables not significantly adding to model and therefore omitted:

Column A: household income, household language;

Column B: maternal age at first live birth, ward type, interview language, household language, lone parenthood, sex of child, ever smoked in pregnancy.

~Other variables significantly predicting:

Column A: number of children in the household, UK country, maternal employment status, gender of child;

Column B: UK country, number of children in the household, mother's employment status, ethnicity.

Source: adapted from Pearce et al. (2008), Tables 3 and 4.

As the table suggests, being completely unimmunized was associated with indicators of disadvantage (Column A). For example, children whose mothers smoked during pregnancy, were lone parents, or were younger than 20 when they were born had higher risks for being unimmunized. However, children whose mothers had high educational qualifications or who were older at the birth of the cohort child (generally an indication of advantage) were also less likely to have been immunized with MMR. A different pattern emerged when comparing those who had received single vaccines to those who had had MMR vaccine (Column B). Predictors of being protected by the single vaccine, which is only available privately and for a fee, were in general associated with better-off families. Single vaccines were used more in families with a high household income and level of maternal education, and an older mother.

Although the commonest reason for not accepting MMR was a conscious decision to refuse it, a significant number of mothers of unimmunized children cited practical reasons for their child not being immunized. This suggests a need for more flexible and accessible immunization services. The complex inequalities in vaccine uptake indicate that information about the advantages of immunization need to be sensitive to the different concerns, questions and beliefs of different groups. Because of the need to ensure herd immunity, tackling low rates of immunization only in some groups is unlikely to protect those living in disadvantage, who remain at the highest risk.

Inequalities in breastfeeding

Breastfeeding provides the optimum nutrition for most babies and protects them from infection, in addition to possible longer-term benefits, including a lower risk of becoming overweight (Gartner et al., 2005). Breastfeeding rates are lower among mothers from disadvantaged groups, increasing health risks for their children (Bolling et al., 2007). However, data from surveys are not usually sufficiently detailed to examine the interrelationships between individual characteristics and breastfeeding. The next section will show how analysis of the MCS has furthered understanding of the relationship between disadvantage and breastfeeding, and how policies and trends in maternal employment and migration may influence inequalities in breastfeeding (and so life-course health) in the future.

At the time the members of the MCS were born (2000 and 2001), the UK government recommended that babies should be breastfed for at least four months. However, analysis of the 18,150 women who were natural mothers of singleton babies in MCS showed that while 70 per cent of mothers had ever put their baby to the breast, only 38 per cent were still being breastfed at four months (Griffiths et al., 2005). These low over-all proportions for breastfeeding mask even lower rates in some groups. Table 1.1.2 shows an analysis of independent socio-economic risk factors for initiating breastfeeding (that is, ever putting the baby to the breast). In addition to assessing the contribution of individual characteristics, the analysis also considered community-level indicators of social advantage, with wards being categorized according to whether or not they were ma-terially advantaged or had high proportions of minority ethnic residents (referred to as 'ethnic wards'). Mothers who were living in advantaged or ethnic wards, those with managerial and professional occupations, and those who were educated to degree level or above were more likely to start breastfeeding than their less advantaged peers. Mothers in couple fami-lies and older mothers were also more likely to start breastfeeding than lone mothers or younger mothers. The risk ratios show that, for example, breastfeeding rates for mothers in couple families would be expected to be 20 per cent higher than rates for lone mothers, even if all other risk factors for breastfeeding (socio-economic status, maternal education and so on) were the same (Griffiths et al., 2005).

Table 1.1.2 also illustrates that mothers from minority ethnic groups were more likely to start breastfeeding than white mothers. Although be-ing a member of a minority ethnic group is often associated with material disadvantage, it seems that this is not accompanied by the low rates of breastfeeding seen among disadvantaged white women. Furthermore, as noted earlier, living in an ethnic ward was associated with an increased rate of starting to breastfeed, this result being demonstrated for both white and minority ethnic women. This suggests that cultural and community factors associated with being from a minority ethnic group may be ex-erting a beneficial influence on the majority white population. Indeed, white women who had a partner of different ethnicity to themselves were 14 per cent more likely to breastfeed than white women with a white partner (Griffiths et al., 2005). Together, these results suggest that peer influences, at personal and community levels, are effective at influencing breastfeeding behaviour and might be a suitable mechanism for develop-ment of policy. Indeed, policies based on neighbourhood renewal, com-munity engagement and the development of social capital (DH, 2003) recognize the power of peer influence, and some health services use peer-support programmes to promote breastfeeding (National Institute for Health and Clinical Excellence, 2008).

The higher rates of breastfeeding among minority ethnic mothers, as well as the apparent breastfeeding-promoting effect of partner and com-munity minority ethnicity for all mothers, are likely to be connected to the preservation of cultural and social attitudes to breastfeeding within minority ethnic groups. Although these may vary by ethnic group, in the

Table 1.1.2 Adjusted risk ratios (RR) and 95 per cent confidence intervals (CI) for initiation of breastfeeding among mothers in England

Measures	Adjusted[a] RR (95% CI)
Ward type	
Disadvantaged	1
Advantaged	1.15 (1.10 to 1.21)
Ethnic	1.11 (1.04 to 1.17)
Ethnic group	
White	1
Other-white	1.24 (1.19 to 1.29)
Mixed	1.45 (1.35 to 1.56)
Indian	1.25 (1.16 to 1.34)
Pakistani	1.27 (1.19 to 1.35)
Bangladeshi	1.56 (1.45 to 1.66)
Black Caribbean	1.57 (1.48 to 1.68)
Black African	1.55 (1.46 to 1.65)
Other ethnic group	1.36 (1.29 to 1.43)
Socio-economic status	
Managerial and professional occupations	1.13 (1.09 to 1.18)
Small employers and own account workers	1.08 (1.04 to 1.13)
Intermediate occupations	1.13 (1.07 to 1.20)
Lower supervisory and technical occupations	1.07 (1.00 to 1.14)
Semi-routine and routine occupations	1
Never worked and long-term unemployed	1.03 (0.97 to 1.09)
Highest academic qualification	
Degree/higher degree	1.39 (1.30 to 1.48)
Diploma in higher education	1.33 (1.25 to 1.42)
A/AS/S levels	1.40 (1.31 to 1.49)
GCSE grades A–C	1.19 (1.12 to 1.27)
GCSE grades D–G	1.11 (1.04 to 1.18)
Other or overseas qualifications	1.22 (1.14 to 1.30)
None of these qualifications	1
Lone-mother status	
Lone mother	1
Non-lone mother	1.20 (1.15 to 1.26)
Age at first ever live birth[b]	1.06 (1.04 to 1.08)
Parity	
Cohort baby not first live born	1
Cohort baby first live born	1.08 (1.05 to 1.11)

Notes
[a]Adjusted for ward type, ethnic group, socio-economic status, academic qualification, lone mother status, age at MCS birth, age at first live birth, parity.
[b]Per five-year increase in maternal age.
Source: adapted from Griffiths et al. (2005), Table 3.

UK, overall they seem to promote breastfeeding. However, after immigration, acculturation – the adoption of health behaviours from the new dominant culture and loss of health behaviours from the original culture – may erode the high rates of breastfeeding among minority ethnic groups. In the MCS, questions were asked of the mothers of the cohort member about their parents' country of birth and how long their family had lived in the UK. This allowed analysis of how indicators of acculturation (for example, whether the mother was an immigrant or was born in the UK) were related to breastfeeding (Hawkins et al., 2008). Although breastfeeding rates vary by ethnic group (as shown earlier), for this analysis, all minority ethnic mothers were considered together, in order to assess the effect of acculturation regardless of ethnicity. First- and second-generation mothers (those who had been born in the UK) were less likely than immigrant mothers to either start breastfeeding or continue to four months (Table 1.1.3). The most pronounced differences were seen for second-generation mothers, who were only half as likely to breastfeed for four months as immigrant mothers. These analyses indicate that the positive breastfeeding patterns among minority ethnic women and communities should be actively protected and supported, because prevalent cultural influences within the UK tend to undermine them (Hawkins et al., 2008).

A major plank in the current government's policies to tackle child poverty is to encourage paid employment for one or both parents (HM Treasury, 2004). For low-income couple families, this often means both parents going to work and in the UK support is provided for lone parents to find employment if their children are under 16. In recent decades, maternal employment has increased rapidly. In 2000, nearly 30 per cent of mothers returned to work by the time their baby was four or five months old (Hamlyn et al., 2002). In 2005, this figure was 13 per cent, but with the percentage on paid or unpaid maternity leave increasing from 22 per cent in 2000 to 43 per cent in 2005 (Bolling et al., 2007). Employment of mothers of children under five years of age has increased from 27 per cent in 1984 to 56 per cent in 2005, with a greater increase among lone parents (ONS, 2006). However, maternal employment in infancy is associated with lower rates of breastfeeding (Bolling et al., 2007). The detailed data on maternal employment and social circumstances in the MCS were used to assess whether breastfeeding is linked to patterns of maternal employment and, if so, whether employment policies might be developed to support breastfeeding among women in paid work.

The analysis was conducted on 6917 white mothers who were employed when the nine-month data collection of MCS was carried out. After adjustment for confounding factors (such as socio-economic position), many features of employment influenced whether a woman continued breastfeeding (Table 1.1.4). Women were more likely to breastfeed for

Table 1.1.3 Adjusted risk ratios (RR) and 95 per cent confidence intervals (CI) for breastfeeding among mothers from minority ethnic groups, according to generational status

Generational status	Breastfeeding initiation		Breastfeeding for at least four months	
	% of participants who breastfed*	Adjusted[‡] RR (95% CI)	% of participants who breastfed*	Adjusted[†] RR (95% CI)
Immigrant	87	1	44	1
First generation	85	0.92 (0.88 to 0.97)	35	0.72 (0.62 to 0.83)
Second generation	83	0.86 (0.75 to 0.99)	26	0.52 (0.30 to 0.89)

Notes

*Weighted percentage.

[†] Adjusted for ethnic group, socio-economic circumstances, family income, highest academic qualification, single motherhood, age at cohort birth, parity.

Source: adapted from Hawkins et al. (2008), Table 3.

Table 1.1.4 Weighted percentages, adjusted risk ratios (RR) and 95 per cent confidence intervals (CI) for breastfeeding for at least four months among British/Irish white employed mothers

	Breastfeeding for at least four months		Adjusted* RR (95% CI)
	n	(weighted %)	
Employment characteristics			
Employment status			
Full time	1787	25	1
Part time	4648	26	1.30 (1.17 to 1.44)
Self-employed	482	41	1.74 (1.46 to 2.07)
Return to employment			
3 months or less	1204	18	0.81 (0.68 to 0.96)
4 months	1475	16	0.74 (0.63 to 0.87)
5 months	1244	22	1
6 months	874	32	1.25 (1.07 to 1.47)
7 months	1031	39	1.53 (1.34 to 1.74)
8 months or more	1064	39	1.54 (1.36 to 1.73)
Number of hours (h) working			
1–10	676	34	1
11–20	2499	25	0.79 (0.70 to 0.90)
21–30	1832	28	0.68 (0.58 to 0.79)
31–40	1578	25	0.63 (0.45 to 0.90)
41+	327	28	0.63 (0.43 to 0.92)
Working atypical hours			
Yes	2931	25	1.05 (0.97 to 1.14)
No	3985	28	1
Working for financial reasons			
Yes	4918	25	0.86 (0.80 to 0.93)
No	1999	32	1
Working because used up maternity leave			
Yes	2148	28	1.01 (0.92 to 1.11)
No	4757	27	1
Employer offers any family-friendly arrangements			
Yes	1004	37	1.14 (1.02 to 1.27)
No	5395	24	1
Employer offers any flexible arrangements			
Yes	5777	27	1.24 (1.00 to 1.55)
No	648	19	1
Number of employees			
Works alone	481	43	1.60 (1.35 to 1.91)
2–24	2256	21	1
25 or more	4163	28	1.15 (1.05 to 1.27)

(continued)

Table 1.1.4   *(Continued)*

	Breastfeeding for at least four months		
	n	(weighted %)	Adjusted* RR (95% CI)
Day care			
Type of day care			
Mother/partner	1869	25	1
Informal	2859	19	0.81 (0.71 to 0.91)
Formal	1969	38	1.07 (0.95 to 1.20)
Maternity leave			
Maternity leave pay			
Statutory Maternity Pay plus additional pay	3275	31	1.13 (1.02 to 1.26)
Statutory Maternity Pay only	2406	23	1
Other pay	173	39	1.27 (0.98 to 1.63)
None	279	28	1.15 (0.93 to 1.42)

Note

*Adjusted for highest academic qualification, socio-economic status, UK country, lone mother status, age at birth of cohort child, age at first live birth, number of children in household and employment status.

Source: adapted from Hawkins et al. (2007), Table 1.

four months if they worked part time or were self-employed (compared to working full time), returned to work after four months, or if they worked fewer hours. They were less likely to breastfeed if they worked atypical hours, returned to work for financial reasons, and did not have access to family-friendly or flexible working arrangements. They were also more likely to breastfeed if they worked alone or in large organizations (25 or more employees) than if they worked in a small organization (2–24 employees). While residual confounding remains possible, these results were robust to adjustment for a range of confounding variables (Hawkins et al., 2007). This suggests that greater use of employment policies such as family-friendly and flexible working might help mothers who choose or are obliged to work to continue to breastfeed. Since the MCS babies were born, maternity leave provision has become more generous. This MCS analysis suggests this change in provision may also promote breastfeeding. However, it also indicates that policies which encourage maternal employment in infancy (even if indirectly) to reduce family poverty may also increase inequalities in breastfeeding. It also illustrates that policies and their resultant changes on families may be both causes of, and solutions to, health inequalities.

Conclusion

A life-course approach to children's health considers not only their health now but the health of the adults they will become. It describes how the different paths through childhood vary by children's social circumstance and how this variation permits or prevents children from accumulating the resources necessary for a healthy, productive and long life. From the overview of data describing UK children's current health and circumstances presented in this chapter, it is apparent that unacceptable variation exists in children's circumstances with consequent inequalities in their current health and likely inequalities in their future adult health. Poorer children are less likely to live to their first birthday than babies born to richer parents (discussed further in Chapter 1.3). And, as they go through their early years, childhood and adolescence, children from families living in disadvantaged circumstances are more likely than their more advantaged peers to be exposed to poverty, poor educational opportunities and a low-quality environment, and to engage in a range of health-related behaviours that are likely to lead to poorer health as they grow up. The detailed examples from the UK's Millennium Cohort Study show the inequalities that are present in the youngest members of our society. Immunization and breastfeeding both promote lifelong health, yet are socially patterned in complex ways, leaving many children without their benefits. However, the analysis also shows the potential for policy and practice to tackle those inequalities, for example, through making services responsive to people's different needs, through building on strengths in communities, and through promoting family-friendly employment policies.

Neil Postman (1982) said that 'Children are a living message we send to a time we will not see'. We need to act swiftly and decisively to ensure that the message we send is a positive one.

Acknowledgments

I would like to thank Richard Jenkins and the Millennium Cohort Study team at the Centre for Longitudinal Studies, Institute of Education, University of London and the Millennium Cohort Study Child Health Group at UCL Institute of Child Health.

Funding statement

This work was undertaken at GOSH/UCL Institute of Child Health which received a proportion of funding from the Department of Health's NIHR Biomedical Research Centres funding scheme. The Centre for Paediatric

Epidemiology and Biostatistics also benefits from funding support from the Medical Research Council in its capacity as the MRC Centre of Epidemiology for Child Health.

References

Batty, G.B. and Leon, D.A. (2002) Socio-economic position and coronary heart disease risk factors in children and young people: evidence from UK epidemiological studies, *European Journal of Public Health*, 12: 263–72.

Bolling, K., Grant, C., Hamlyn, B. et al. (2007) *Infant Feeding Survey 2005*. Leeds: The Information Centre.

Brewer M., Muriel A., Phillips D. and Sibieta, L. (2008) *Poverty and Inequality in the UK: 2008*. London: Institute for Fiscal Studies.

British Medical Association (2006) *Child and Adolescent Mental Health: A Guide for Healthcare Professionals*. London: BMA.

Brodersen, N.H., Steptoe, A., Boniface, R. et al. (2007) Trends in physical activity and sedentary behaviour in adolescence: ethnic and socioeconomic differences, *British Journal of Sports Medicine*, 41:140–4.

Cawson, P., Wattam, C., Brooker, S. et al. (2000) *Child Maltreatment in the United Kingdom: A Study of the Prevalence of Abuse and Neglect*. London: NSPCC.

Centre for Longitudinal Studies (2008) *Millennium Cohort Study*. Available at: http://www.cls.ioe.ac.uk/studies.asp?section=000100020001.

Craig, R. and Mindell, J. (2008) *Health Survey for England 2006: Cardiovascular Disease and Risk Factors. Summary of Key Findings*. Leeds: The Information Centre.

Department for Children, Schools and Families (DCSF) (2008) *Statistical First Release. Outcome Indicators for Children Looked After: Twelve Months to 30 September 2007, England*. London: DCSF.

Department for Communities and Local Government (DCLG) (2008) *English House Condition Survey 2006 Headline Report*. London: DCLG.

Department for Work and Pensions (DWP) (2006) *Making a Difference: Tackling Poverty – a Progress Report*. London: DWP.

Department for Work and Pensions (DWP) (2007) *Households Below Average Income (HBAI) 1994/95–2005/06 (Revised)*. Available at: http://www.dwp.gov.uk/asd/hbai/hbai2006/contents.asp.

Department of Health (DH) (2003) *Tacking Health Inequalities: A Programme for Action*. London: DH.

Department of Health (DH) (2008) *Tackling Health Inequalities: 2007 Status Report on the Programme for Action*. London: DH.

Dolk, H., Pattenden, S. and Johnson, A. (2001) Cerebral palsy, low birth-weight and socio-economic deprivation: inequalities in a major cause of childhood disability, *Paediatric and Perinatal Epidemiology*, 15: 359–63.

Douglas-Hall, A. and Chau, M. (2008) *Basic Facts about Low-income Children: Birth to Age 18*. Available at: http://www.nccp.org/publications/pdf/text_845.pdf.

Ferguson, B., Merrick, D., Evans, S. et al. (2006) *Indications of Public Health in the English Regions. 5: Child Health*. York: Association of Public Health Observatories.

Fuller, E. (2007) *Smoking, Drinking and Drug Use among Young People in England in 2006*. Leeds: The Information Centre.

Gartner, L.M., Morton, J., Lawrence, R.A. et al. (2005) Breastfeeding and the use of human milk, *Pediatrics*, 115: 496–506.

Graham, H. and Power, C. (2004) Childhood disadvantage and health inequalities: a framework for policy based on lifecourse research. *Child: Care, Health and Development*, 30: 671–8.

Griffiths, L.J., Tate, A.R., Dezateux, C. et al. (2005) The contribution of parental and community ethnicity to breastfeeding practices: evidence from the Millenium Cohort Study, *International Journal of Epidemiology*, 34: 1378–86.

Hamlyn, B., Brooker, S., Oleinikova, K. et al. (2002) *Infant Feeding 2000. A Survey Conducted on Behalf of the Department of Health, the Scottish Executive, the National Assembly for Wales and the Department of Health, Social Services and Public Safety in Northern Ireland*. London: The Stationery Office.

Hawkins, S.S., Griffiths, L.J., Dezateux, C. et al. (2007) The impact of maternal employment on breast-feeding duration in the UK Millennium Cohort Study, *Public Health Nutrition*, 10: 891–6.

Hawkins, S.S., Lamb, K., Cole, T.J. et al. (2008) Influence of moving to the UK on maternal health behaviours: prospective cohort study, *British Medical Journal*, 336: 1052–5.

HM Treasury (2004) *Child Poverty Review*. Norwich: The Stationery Office.

Kuh, D. and Ben-Shlomo, Y. (1997) *A Life Course Approach to Chronic Disease*. Oxford: Oxford University Press.

Lake, J.K., Power, C. and Cole, T.J. (1997) Child to adult body mass index in the 1958 British birth cohort: associations with parental obesity, *Archives of Disease in Childhood*, 77: 376–81.

Li, J., McMurray, A. and Stanley, F. (2008) Modernity's paradox and the structural determinants of child health and well-being, *Health Sociology Review*, 17: 64–77.

Lobstein, T., Baur, L. and Uauy, R. (2004) Obesity in children and young people: a crisis in public health, *Obesity Review*, 5(suppl 1): 4–85.

London Health Observatory (2007) *Born Equal? A Briefing on Inequalities in Infant Mortality in London*. London: London Health Observatory.

McDowell, M.M., Wang, C-Y. and Kennedy-Stephenson, J. (2008) *NCHS Data Brief, No.5, April 2008. Breastfeeding in the United States: Findings from the National Health and Nutrition Examination Surveys, 1999–2006.* Available at: http://www.cdc.gov/nchs/data/databriefs/db05.pdf.

Meltzer, H., Gatward, R., Goodman, R. et al. (2000) *The Mental Health of Children and Adolescents in Great Britain: Summary Report*. London: The Stationery Office.

Middleton, E. and Baker, D. (2003) Comparison of social distribution of immunisation with measles, mumps, and rubella vaccine, England, 1991–2001, *British Medical Journal*, 326: 854.

National Institute for Health and Clinical Excellence (2008) *Improving the Nutrition of Pregnant and Breastfeeding Mothers and Children in Low-income Households. NICE Public Health Guidance 11.* London: National Institute for Health and Clinical Excellence.

Nessa, N. and Gallagher, J. (2004) Diet, nutrition, dental health and exercise, in Office for National Statistics (ed.) *The Health of Children and Young People*. London: Office for National Statistics.

Office for National Statistics (2006) *Work and Family: Half of Mums of under 5's Are in Employment*. Available at: http://www.statistics.gov.uk/cci/nugget.asp?id=1655.

Olshansky, S.J., Passaro, D.J., Hershow, R.C. et al. (2005) A potential decline in life expectancy in the United States in the 21st century, *New England Journal of Medicine*, 352: 1138–45.

Parsons, T.J., Power, C., Logan, S. et al. (1999) Childhood predictors of adult obesity: a systematic review. *International Journal of Obesity*, 23(suppl 8): S1–S107.

Pearce, A., Law, C., Elliman, D. et al. (2008) Factors associated with uptake of measles, mumps, and rubella vaccine (MMR) and use of single antigen vaccines in a contemporary UK cohort: prospective cohort study, *British Medical Journal*, 336, 754–7.

Pickett, K.E. and Wilkinson, R.G. (2007) Child wellbeing and income inequality in rich societies: ecological cross sectional study, *British Medical Journal*, 335: 1080–5.

Postman, N. (1982) *The Disappearance of Childhood*. New York: Delacorte Press.

Shrewsbury, V. and Wardle, J. (2008) Socioeconomic status and adiposity in childhood: a systematic review of cross-sectional studies 1990–2005, *Obesity*, 16:275–84.

Singh, G.K. and Kogan, M.D. (2007) Persistent socioeconomic disparities in infant, neonatal, and postneonatal mortality rates in the United States, 1969–2001. *Pediatrics*, 119:e928–39.

Spencer, N. (2003) *Weighing the Evidence: How Is Birthweight Determined?* Abingdon: Radcliffe.

UNICEF Innocenti Research Centre (2007) *An Overview of Child Well-being in Rich Countries: A Comprehensive Assessment of the Lives and Well-being of Children and Adolescents in the Economically Advanced Nations.* Florence: UNICEF.

Wakefield, A., Murch, S., Anthony, A. et al. (1998) Ileal-lymphoid-nodular hyperplasia, non-specific colitis, and pervasive developmental disorder in children, *Lancet*, 351: 637–41.

World Health Organization (WHO) Commission on Social Determinants of Health (2008) *Closing the Gap in a Generation: Health Equity Through Action on the Social Determinants of Health.* Geneva: WHO.

1.2 Life-course influences on health at older ages

Mel Bartley and David Blane

Introduction

Health inequalities at older ages are little studied, compared with those during childhood and the years of working life. This is true both in the UK and internationally. For example, in Britain's most recent *Decennial Supplement on Occupational Mortality*, only 5 of the 128 tables and only 2 of the 97 figures refer to social class differences in all-cause mortality at ages over 65 years (Drever and Whitehead, 1997). To some extent, this relative neglect is caused by doubts about the applicability to retired people of occupation-based measures of social class, although the need to solve such problems is becoming urgent because life expectancy in middle age is increasing, with the result that a growing proportion of all deaths occur at ages after retirement from paid employment.

Evidence for England and Wales illustrates that although social class differences in mortality are found long after retirement age (Table 1.2.1), they are widest among young people and narrow with increasing age (Table 1.2.2). However, because deaths cluster at older ages, these relatively modest inequalities are associated with a large number of deaths. Studies of health inequalities have moved during the past 10 years from description to explanation; and interest in the life-course perspective has grown as part of this process, not least because the prevalent causes of death at older ages have aetiologies and natural histories that stretch back decades.

The life-course approach to health and health inequalities brings together social science, biological science and longitudinal methods of study and analysis. We know that social processes are the drivers of the relationship between the social and the biological, because of the existence of social class differences in health (Drever and Whitehead, 1997; Khaw, 1999). Social class is an historically specific product of human organization, yet somehow it gets into the molecules, cells and tissues of the body to produce social class differences in life expectancy and cause of death. Consequently, a key question explored by life-course research is: how does the social become biological? Our attempt to answer the question

Table 1.2.1   All-cause mortality per 1000 person, years by age at death and Civil Service grade during working life, England and Wales

	Age at death	
	65–69 years	*70–89 years*
Administrative	17.4	32.6
Professional and executive	17.3	44.8
Clerical	26.7	65.4
Other	32.1	70.9

Source: adapted from Marmot and Shipley (1996), Table 1 .

draws on British studies. The chapter discusses evidence from four key methods for studying life-course influences on health at older ages, with sections looking in turn at birth cohort studies, cross-sectional analyses, the discovery and investigation of historical records (called 'epidemiological archaeology') and longitudinal studies. We set the scene for these sections by briefly discussing models of social and aetiological processes and different methods of study.

Social and aetiological processes

Social processes

The main social process is the accumulation of advantages or disadvantages (Blane, 2006). Advantages and disadvantages tend to cluster cross-sectionally, so that the same people who endure disadvantage in the occupational sphere (musculo-skeletal, physico-chemical and psycho-social hazards) tend, as a consequence of low pay, to endure also disadvantage in

Table 1.2.2   Life expectancy (years) by Registrar General social class, England and Wales, 1987–91

	Social classes I & II	*Social classes IV & V*	*Difference I & II v. IV & V*
Men:			
At age 15	60.5	55.8	4.7
At age 65	15.0	12.4	2.6
Women:			
At age 15	65.8	62.5	3.3
At age 65	18.7	16.7	2.0

Source: adapted from Hattersley (1997), Table 6.1.

the domestic sphere (residential crowding and damp, local atmospheric pollution, poor diet). Conversely, those who enjoy occupational advantage (no hazards, flexible working, long holidays) tend also to enjoy residential advantage (space, quiet, safety, varied diet, local green space). These advantages or disadvantages also tend to accumulate longitudinally. A disadvantaged childhood militates against adolescent educational success and in favour of adult low-skilled labour, which leads to reliance at older ages on the minimum state pension; and, conversely, an affluent childhood encourages adolescent educational success and adult professional employment, which leads to an occupational pension at older ages.

Jerry Morris, a leading British epidemiologist, has quantified a central aspect of this process; namely, income. Using the best scientific evidence to identify the requirements for a healthy life, he has costed these necessities for a single young man and for a retired single person and couple (Morris et al., 2000, 2007). The minimum income for healthy living for a young man was more than the statutory minimum wage for 40 hours per week and considerably more than welfare benefits if unemployed. Of greater relevance to the present chapter, the minimum income for healthy living for retired people was greater than the pension credit guarantee and considerably more than the state pension. Morris's costings assume that his subjects live the lives of paragons, so it is reasonable to assume that many older people week after week, on a long-term basis, lack the money to live a healthy life.

In relation to the minimum cost of healthy living for older people, *how the social becomes biological* can be illustrated by two pieces of work. Poor-quality housing within Britain tends to be located in areas where the climate is most demanding in terms of cold and wet (called the 'inverse housing law' and discussed in more detail later in the chapter). Residence in poor-quality housing in a region with severe climate has been shown to be associated with reduced lung function (Blane et al., 2000) and raised diastolic and systolic blood pressure (Mitchell et al., 2002). The inverse housing law affects particularly older people, because they often lack the money to renovate their homes to a standard that ensures protection against the local climate and because older people are more vulnerable to air pollution because of their age-related respiratory and cardiovascular decline.

Aetiological processes

The effect at older ages of air pollution and the inverse housing law will tend to accumulate on top of damage from earlier in life – for example, repeated respiratory tract infections during childhood due to residential crowding, local atmospheric pollution during adolescent play and sports and tobacco smoking and occupational fumes and dusts during the years of working life (Mann et al., 1992). In this case, the social process of accumulation matches the aetiological process by which serial damage accumulates over the life course, which may explain why social class differences in death due to diseases of the lung tend to be wider than for other causes of death.

In addition to accumulation, two other aetiological processes relevant to understanding life-course influences on health have been described: biological programming (Barker, 1994) and pathways (Power and Hertzman, 1997). In biological programming, sub-optimal fetal organ development predisposes to adult disease. Sub-optimal fetal lung development, for example, predisposes to adult chronic obstructive pulmonary disease; sub-optimal foetal kidney development to adult hypertension; sub-optimal fetal pancreatic development to adult diabetes; and so forth. In the pathway model, early experiences set individuals on social pathways into adolescence and adulthood – on educational pathways and occupational careers for example – which then impact on their future circumstances and their future health (discussed in the Hilary Graham's introductry chapter and Chapter 1.1). The pathways that people follow influence the health risks to which they are exposed. For example, highly educated women are at increased risk of breast cancer because prolonged education and establishing a career (social process) delivers a woman to a late first pregnancy, which is the aetiologically important event for breast cancer risk. Although the distinction between these three models of life-course aetiology is useful, they can be difficult to separate empirically (Hallqvist et al., 2004) and theoretically (Blane, Netuveli and Stone, 2007).

Birth cohort studies

Of the four birth cohort studies in the UK (1946, 1958, 1970, Millennium), only the first two are aged sufficiently to be relevant to the present chapter. Of these, only the first (the 1946 birth cohort Study) is approaching the life-course stage where most morbidity and mortality now are concentrated. Nevertheless, even if, in relation to ageing, the future insights from the birth cohort studies promise more than has been achieved so far, their findings about approaching early old age are unique, because they are based on prospective life-course data, free of the potential biases of recalled information.

National Survey of Health and Development (1946 birth cohort)

The oldest of the British birth cohort studies, the *National Survey of Health and Development*, was started in 1946, a time of major social and policy change in the UK. The legislation establishing the National Health Service had been passed, although universal free health care was not a reality until 1948. However, for the great majority of their lives, the members of this cohort were among the first worldwide to be covered by health care that did not require payment at the time of use.

The motivation behind the study is still reflected in the composition of the sample. One policy concern at the time was the apparent failure of the middle classes to reproduce. Consequently, the sample was biased towards more affluent families, with only 1 in 4 children of working-class families included. All children of non-manual and agricultural families plus this sub-group of children of manual families have been followed up 21 times, the latest being at age 53 years.

In 1946, the British social structure was also far different to what it is today, in that the great majority of people earned their living from some kind of manual work. Smoking was not yet regarded as a health hazard, so we will never know which members of this cohort's mothers smoked during their pregnancies. However, most of the important findings of the study as it went along could not possibly have been anticipated. The post-war economy in Britain, as in many other nations, made it possible for a far higher proportion of the male population to be employed than had been the case for many decades (the First World War having been followed by successive crises of unemployment). Nationalization of the mines, railways, shipyards and steel manufacture resulted in steady work for large numbers of men who may have acquired a high degree of skill during their working lives, but were not required to have left school with any qualifications. A massive programme of house building added to these important social changes. The very existence of a Welfare State created large numbers of white-collar jobs in the administration of social services, education, local government, housing and health services. A vacuum opened up in the occupational structure that 'sucked' many people away from manual backgrounds into these middle-class jobs.

As we come to study ageing in the 1946 birth cohort, therefore, we need to be aware that the life experiences of these people have been very different from those of previous ones, and of those that followed. Upward social mobility, from manual to non-manual work, was higher than at any time before or since. The proportion of people who married and had children was also greater, with younger ages at marriage and first childbirth.

Research using these data to the present has concentrated on relatively simple measures of socio-economic disadvantage in childhood, as well as psychological and biological variables, in relation to health at older ages and to mortality. These studies have provided remarkable examples of long-range life-course effects over 50 years or more. Social and economic disadvantage in childhood (defined in terms of the father's occupation) predicted shorter height, which is a risk factor for heart and lung disease, at age 36 years (Kuh and Wadsworth, 1989). Disability at age 43 years was related to ill health in childhood and to socio-economic disadvantage at all phases of the life course (Kuh et al., 1994). Childhood illness was, moreover, more likely to predict adult disability in those with a less favourable socio-economic life history. Childhoood disadvantage, as measured by manual social class of the father, was found to be related to lower levels of physical function half a century later in male study participants at age 53 years (Guralnik et al., 2006).

Studies using 1946 cohort data have begun to test some of the hypotheses proposed in the previous section, although rather less research has focused on complex combinations of social and physical exposures. Educational success seems to have been one of the important pathways between early social circumstances and health in later middle age. Paternal social class is strongly related to educational success in this, as in all other studies. Cohort members with only low levels of education were more affected in middle age by various risk factors for heart disease such as high blood pressure, overweight and high blood fats (Langenberg et al., 2006). Cognitive function ('intelligence') is related to many aspects of health in this cohort, raising the issue of whether more intelligent participants, in adult life, manage to look after their own health better. One of the most important papers covering the topic shows that cognitive function at age 8 years was related to the risk of death up to age 54 years. However, what seemed to be important for life expectancy was the fact that the better educated obtained better paid and more privileged employment, rather than any behavioural factors such as smoking or exercise (Kuh et al., 2004). In this way, the founding member of the family of British birth cohort studies directs us towards paying attention to the ways in which pathways through the social structure begin to be shaped very early in life, and how these pathways involve combinations of exposures to risk and protective factors. It also highlights the extent to which social pathways and their implications for health depend on the social structure itself, in this case, the availability of safe, well-paid employment.

As one might expect from a study funded entirely by the UK's Medical Research Council, the 1946 cohort has focused rather more closely on how biological factors such as birthweight, growth in infancy, breast feeding and childhood illness relate to health at older ages. However, the increasing levels of interest in early childhood growth should be regarded as an example of what is made possible by inter-disciplinary work. Growth in humans up to around age seven years, before the pubertal growth spurt, is thought to be influenced by the quality of the child's emotional environment. These ideas are based on work with animals, in which denying access to maternal nurturance (such as licking and grooming in rats) has long been known to reduce growth in the offspring. Slower growth can be measured easily, but it is regarded as an indicator of the development of systems in the brain, which develops at great speed in these early years, and which later will regulate responses to fear and stress. In adulthood, individuals who grew slowly as children are often found to have shorter legs relative to their height (Gunnell et al., 1998; Li et al., 2007). The 1946 cohort study has been one of the first to begin to test relationships between slower growth in early childhood, shorter leg length, and risk factors for later-life diseases such as heart attacks (Wadsworth et al., 2002; Langenberg et al., 2005). The inter-relationships of early life socio-emotional experience, child growth, adult height and adult health are now increasingly being explored, with results that promise to increase our understanding of complex life-course influences (Gunnell et al., 2003). Future research will greatly improve the understanding of those who plan and deliver services and products to older people.

National Child Development Study (1958 birth cohort)

The second of the British birth cohort studies, the *National Child Development Study*, began in 1958. It took all births in a single week of March 1958, and was initially intended to be a study of perinatal health, that is, the health of babies from just before to just after their birth. The information produced was so valuable that decisions were taken to continue following up the study participants; further studies were done when they were aged 7, 11, 16, 23 and 33 years. At age 45 years, a biomedical component was added, in which participants gave blood samples and did various medical tests, with a further survey at age 50 years.

The social and economic context through which the 1958 birth cohort passed was somewhat different to that of the 1946 cohort, although their birth dates are only 12 years apart. The greatest difference was the arrival of deindustrialization, beginning in the late 1970s. The stable jobs in industry available to 16-year-old school leavers in 1962 were still there when the 1958 cohort reached 16 in 1974, but not for very long. Members of the 1958 cohort who left school at the earliest possible age, without qualifications, were in fact at an advantage compared to their peers who went to university. They entered a 'post-war, full-employment' labour market and at first experienced little unemployment. By the time those who stayed in education were looking for jobs, the situation was changing rapidly. However, although those who stayed longer in education were initially at greater risk of unemployment, by the end of the 1980s, their less educated peers had caught up with them and surpassed them as industrial jobs dried up. Possibly as a result of this growing economic insecurity, members of the 1958 cohort were likely to marry and have children quite a lot later than the 1946 cohort, and far more of them remained unmarried and childless.

Participants in the 1958 cohort study were last surveyed at age 50, which is the earliest age when issues around 'ageing' are usually thought to arise. However, as with the 1946 cohort, it can be seen that, even by the medical screening at age 45 years, health functioning was poorer among those with the most disadvantaged life histories (Power et al., 2007; Strachan et al., 2007). Generalized pain, anxiety and depression, hearing problems, being overweight and having high blood pressure and poorer lung function were more prevalent in those born into disadvantaged social circumstances, and highest in those who had continued into a disadvantaged adulthood. This kind of adverse life history was also linked to a number of heart disease risk factors such as high levels of low-density lipoprotein (LDL) – often known as 'bad cholesterol' – and other blood fats (triglycerides) (Power et al., 2007). Further evidence on the relationship of long-term social adversity to health in middle age showed it was possible to compute a 'social disadvantage score' across the life course, according to the number of times a study participant had been in a less advantaged situation at birth and ages 23 and 43 years. These scores at age 45 years were found to predict three measures of inflammatory processes, which in turn predict longer-term health risks (Tabassum et al., 2008).

As yet, disability has not been studied in the 1958 cohort. However, in view of the striking class differences in chronic conditions, disability and health functioning problems at age 53 years in the 1946 cohort, this will prove to be an important next step in studies of health across the life course. Other work that remains to be done as these cohorts move from middle to early old age include investigation of the health effects of specific forms of disadvantage which tend to accumulate over time such as poor housing, polluted areas and work hazards.

Cross-sectional studies

Cross-sectional studies lack the time dimension, which makes it impossible to demonstrate which variable in a relationship, say between social conditions and health, came first. As cause must precede effect, causality in a cross-sectional study may be inferred or reasoned, but it can not be demonstrated.

Three British studies, which were mentioned previously, can be used to illustrate the material context of health, in terms of: (a) the minimum income required by a retired couple to purchase the necessities of life, as identified by the best current scientific evidence; (b) the respiratory and cardiovascular consequences of residential accommodation which provides inadequate protection against local weather conditions; (c) the estimated number of deaths due to acute air pollution episodes – these deaths will be on top of the effects of exposure to chronic air pollution. The social process of the accumulation of advantage or disadvantage indicates that disadvantage in these three areas of life will tend to cluster in the same individuals and that such exposures will tend to accumulate longitudinally.

Minimum income for healthy living: retired couple

Jerry Morris and his colleagues (2007) used the latest biomedical and social research to identify the personal requirements for health and well-being of a retired couple. Their diet was specified to meet the daily energy requirements of a moderately active man and woman aged 75–84 years, their basic nutrient requirements such as vitamins and internationally accepted dietary recommendations on fruit, vegetables and oily fish. This diet cost £63.70 (itemized costs per week for couple at April 2005 values). Their physical activity was specified to include dynamic aerobic exercise, activity against resistance to build muscle mass and exercises to strengthen the ankles for balance (cost £4.10). Their housing was specified to be safe, warm and comfortable (cost £39.48 excluding council tax, rent and mortgage payments). Their medical care included ophthalmic services, dental care and over-the-counter medicines (cost £4.00). Their social requirements were specified to meet the needs for psycho-social relations, social inclusion and active minds (cost £31.10) as well as the presentation of self, to allow them to *appear in public without shame* (cost £37.40). A further £12.30 was added for inefficiencies and emergencies. The total minimum income for healthy living of a retired couple was £192.10 per week at April 2005 prices (equivalent to £208.00 at April 2007 prices).

These costings are conservative. They heat the home for only nine hours per day. They allow only £448.00 per year for maintenance and repair of housing structure. They exclude the cost of taking part in activities such as college extramural classes. They are calculated for those without significant defined disability; the approximately 40 per cent of those aged 65 years plus who are disabled are likely to require additional income to achieve a comparable standard of living. Nevertheless, at April 2007 prices per week, this conservative total (£208.00) exceeds the State Pension for a couple (£139.60) and their Pension Credit Guarantee (£181.70). In other words, each week of their lives a pensioner couple will receive £26.30 less than they need as the minimum income for healthy living; or £68.40 less, if they do not apply for the means-tested Pension Credit Guarantee.

Inverse housing law

The *inverse housing law* refers to the mismatch between climate demand and housing quality. Most areas of Britain that experience poor climate, as measured by low temperature and high rainfall, are characterized also by poor-quality housing, judged by the following indicators: residential locality, tenure, crowding, outdoor toilet, sole use of basic facilities, temperature in living room and indoor carbon monoxide levels. The areas which combine harsh climate and poor housing include Scotland, most of Wales, most of north east England and the areas around Leeds, Manchester and Birmingham; elsewhere harsh climate is compensated by good housing or poor housing is compensated by good climate or both climate and housing are good (Blane et al., 2000). The issue is of particular relevance to health at older ages because some older people lack the funds (as discussed earlier) to maintain and repair their homes, to improve them in relation to, for example, heat insulation and to pay heating bills.

Excess winter mortality in Britain is higher than in other European countries; and most of these excess deaths are at older ages and attributed to cardio-respiratory disease. Research on the inverse housing law has demonstrated two possible mechanisms. In relation to respiratory disease (Blane et al., 2000), the component of housing quality that refers to its physical characteristics and, plausibly, its ability to protect against damp and cold, was defined as *stock quality*. Poor stock quality was measured in terms of outdoor toilet, shared use of basic facilities, low living room temperature and high indoor carbon monoxide level. Stock quality predicted lung function[1] independently of climate, social class and the main potential confounders (tobacco smoking and bronchodilator use), with a statistically significant interaction term for climate by housing stock. The association between stock quality and lung function was strongest among those resident in the worst quarter of the climate distribution. Consequently, on the balance of probabilities, the inverse housing law in this data set (*Health and Lifestyle Survey*) affected respiratory health. Second, in relation to cardiovascular disease (Mitchell et al., 2002), living in poor housing, measured again as *stock quality*, in an area with harsh climate, defined as more than the average number of days per month with ground frost, was associated, after control for potential confounders (age, sex, body mass index, alcohol consumption, ambient temperature, tobacco smoking, anti-hypertensive medication) with an increased risk of diastolic and, more modestly, systolic hypertension. Once again, on the balance of probabilities, the inverse housing law in this data set affected cardiovascular health.

Air pollution

A government committee estimated the number of deaths in Britain associated with acute air pollution episodes. The committee was reluctant to say that pollution caused these deaths, but nevertheless judged it likely that 'the associations are causal' (DH, 1998: 2). It stressed that 'many of the deaths associated with days of higher air pollution are in the elderly and sick' (DH, 1998: 3). Also, in its view 'the overall impacts' of acute episodes and long-term exposure 'may be substantially greater than those we have as yet been able to quantify' (DH, 1998: 3). In other words, their estimates are probably causal, differentially affect older people and are conservative because they ignore long-term effects.

The number of deaths affected by PM_{10} small particulate matter[2] and sulphur dioxide air pollution was estimated only for the urban areas of Britain. In the case of PM_{10} pollution, the number of deaths from all causes brought forward each year was estimated as 8100; the comparable figure for sulphur dioxide was 3500. The number of deaths affected by ozone air pollution was estimated in both urban and rural areas of Britain during the summer months only. The number of deaths from all causes brought forward each year by ozone pollution was estimated as 12,500. Although the committee considered it 'unwise' (DH, 1998: 59), these numbers of deaths can be summed to 24,100 per year, most of which occur among older people, because of their age-related impaired lung function and their higher prevalence of chronic obstructive airway disease and ischaemic heart disease; with, in addition, a large but unknown number of deaths caused by the effects of long-term exposure to air pollution.

Combined effects

Finally, it is important to note that the same individuals are likely to have less than the minimum income for healthy living, suffer from the inverse housing law and have a level of cardio-respiratory impairment which makes them vulnerable to acute air pollution episodes. Further, these same individuals are likely to have had disadvantaged life trajectories prior to early old age (Berney et al., 2000). It is out of such life-course and contemporaneous processes, each perhaps of modest impact on their own, that social class differences in the health of older people are formed.

Epidemiological archaeology

Epidemiological archaeology is the term given to the discovery and investigation of historical records and surveys, often ones that have been long forgotten. It involves unearthing social surveys, particularly those which collected biomedical measurements, and tracing the study participants to their present-day locations in order to resurvey those who are willing to volunteer. The method can include collecting information retrospectively on the period between the original and present-day surveys, perhaps using a lifegrid (Blane, 1996; Berney and Blane 1997) or event history calendar. One study will suffice to illustrate this approach to studying life-course influences on health at older ages.

The Boyd Orr study (named after John Boyd Orr, the first scientist to demonstrate a link between poverty, poor diet and ill health) was set up in the late 1930s as a study of childhood dietary conditions and health in Britain. Surviving members of the study were recontacted by postal questionnaire in the mid-1990s, when a small stratified random sample was selected for interview, including a lifegrid to collect retrospective information about the interviewee's life between 1930s and 1990s, and for anthropometric and physiological measurement.

The full Boyd Orr data set and its lifegrid sub-sample have been used to examine several aspects of life at older ages, including diet (Maynard et al., 2005, 2006), quality of life (Blane et al., 2004; Wiggins et al., 2004) and health (Blane et al., 1998, 1999; Berney et al., 2000; Holland et al., 2000; Montgomery et al., 2000).

The analyses of health at older ages illustrate some of the social and aetiological life-course processes discussed earlier in the chapter. Child growth, as measured by pre-pubertal height in 1937–8 conditioned on adult height in 1997–8, was considered to mark a *critical period* for the development of the brain receptors that control the response to stress, with high levels of psycho-social stress during childhood leading to both stunted child growth, which can be masked by later catch-up growth, and over-production of brain stress receptors, which mis-sets the adult stress response and predisposes to adult hypertension (Montgomery et al., 2000). Being raised in a household characterized by high psycho-social stress is also part of a life trajectory where disadvantage *accumulates*, so those who are shortest in childhood are most likely to be exposed to occupational stress during adulthood (Holland et al., 2000). The processes of critical period and accumulation *interact*, so that blood pressure in early old age of slow-growing children is raised further if, during adulthood, they are exposed to occupational stress (Montgomery et al., 2000).

Interestingly, when compared with health, other dimensions of life at older ages are less influenced by events and circumstances from earlier in the life course. Vegetable consumption during childhood influences diet in early old age, but most other influences are contemporaneous (Maynard et al., 2006). Similarly, quality of life at older ages may be influenced by comparatively recent events during labour market exit (Blane et al., 2004), but the main influences are contemporaneous and cross-sectional (Wiggins et al., 2004).

Longitudinal studies

The *English Longitudinal Study of Ageing* (Marmot et al., 2003; Banks et al., 2006, 2008) is a major new source of information on people aged 50 years and older in England, including information on their wealth (that is, their financial assets, physical and housing assets, but not pensions). Among its findings are that wealth is a more powerful predictor of mortality risk after retirement than social class, as measured by occupation (Nazroo et al., 2008) and that wealth after retirement predicts the onset over a four-year period of impairments in gait speed, activities of daily living, motor skills and mobility (Breeze and Lang, 2008).

The *English Longitudinal Study of Ageing* (ELSA) is part of a family of studies that includes the *Health and Retirement Study* (HRS) in the USA and the *Study of Health, Ageing and Retirement in Europe* (SHARE) covering around 20 countries of mainland Europe. As yet these studies are young, so their prospective longitudinal data are of modest duration, but both ELSA and SHARE are collecting life-course retrospective data by lifegrid (event history calendar), which means that life-course studies will become possible in the future. In the meanwhile, ELSA data have shown that functional limitation, rather than the presence of disease, is the more important predictor of quality of life at older ages (Netuveli et al., 2005); that this relationship is independent of potential psychological confounders (Blane et al., 2008); that efforts to improve quality of life in early old age need to address financial hardship, functionally limiting disease, lack of at least one trusting relationship and inability to move out of a disliked neighbourhood (Netuveli et al., 2006); and that quality of life in early old age is graded stepwise by social class, with the difference between the extremes of the social hierarchy of a comparable size to the difference between not having a long-standing illness and having a limiting long-standing illness (Blane, Netuveli and Bartley 2007).

The *British Household Panel Survey* (BHPS) is a second UK longitudinal data set which has collected information from older people. BHPS is an annual panel survey and, as it started a decade before ELSA, longitudinal analyses of longer duration already are possible. Netuveli and colleagues (2008), for example, used data from each wave of annual data collection between 1991 and 2004 to examine resilience at older ages, which they defined as bouncing back after adversity. The adversities examined were the onset of functionally-limiting illness, loss of marriage partner and transition into poverty; with bouncing-back operationalized as a mental health score on the GHQ-12 measure which one year after the onset of adversity had returned to its pre-adversity level. The resilient were found more likely to have high social support than their non-resilient peers, but otherwise were not different socio-economically. High social support was associated with resilience only if it was present before and at the time of adversity, when it increased the likelihood of resilience by 40–60 per cent compared with those with low social support; high social support initiated after adversity did not confer resilience (Netuveli et al., 2008).

Conclusion

The chapter's title, 'Life-Course Influences on Health at Older Ages', begs the question of what is meant by health. If health is equated with physical well-being, then the birth cohort studies have demonstrated the long-term effects on health in middle age of childhood circumstances and their accumulation with circumstances during early adulthood. The products of epidemiological archaeology, like the Boyd Orr cohort, added to these insights by demonstrating how critical periods during childhood can accumulate with circumstances during adulthood and interact to affect health during early old age. On the other hand, if the definition of health is broadened to include determinants of health, like diet, and aspects of mental well-being, like quality of life and resilience, then life-course influences appear weaker, with the main influences being contemporaneous. Perhaps one way of trying to summarize the patterns emerging from research to date is to say that the past is written into the body while the present shapes behaviour and reactions to life.

Notes

1. Lung function was measured in the standard way as the deviation of the observed FEV_1/FVC ratio from the ratio expected in healthy subjects on the basis of their age and height.
2. PM_{10} is a measure of the size of particulate matter; finer particles are generally more health-damaging than coarser particles.

Acknowledgments

Work for this chapter was part of the scientific programme of the ESRC International Centre for Life Course Studies in Society and Health, grant no RES-596-28-0001.

References

Banks, J., Breeze, E., Lessof, C. and Nazroo, J. (eds) (2006) *Retirement, Health and Relationships of the Older Population in England: The 2004 English Longitudinal Study of Ageing*. London: Institute of Fiscal Studies.

Banks, J., Breeze, E., Lessof, C. and Nazroo, J. (eds) (2008) *Living in the 21st Century: Older People in England: The 2006 English Longitudinal Study of Ageing*. London: Institute of Fiscal Studies.

Barker, D. (1994) *Mothers, Babies and Disease in Later Life.* London: BMJ.

Berney, L. and Blane, D. (1997) Collecting retrospective data: accuracy of recall after 50 years judged against historical records, *Social Science and Medicine.* 45: 1519–25.

Berney, L., Blane, D., Davey Smith, G. et al. (2000) Socioeconomic measures in early old age as indicators of previous lifetime exposure to environmental health hazards, *Sociology of Health and Illness*, 22: 415–30.

Blane, D. (1996) Collecting retrospective data: development of a reliable method and a pilot study of its use, *Social Science and Medicine*, 42: 751–7.

Blane, D. (2006) The life course, the social gradient and health, in M. Marmot and R. Wilkinson (eds) *Social Determinants of Health.* Oxford: Oxford University Press.

Blane, D., Bartley, M. and Mitchell, R. (2000) The 'Inverse Housing Law' and respiratory health, *Journal of Epidemiology and Community Health*, 54: 745–9.

Blane, D., Berney, L., Davey Smith, G., Gunnell, D. and Holland, P. (1999) Reconstructing the life course: a 60 year follow-up study based on the Boyd Orr cohort, *Public Health*, 113: 117–24.

Blane, D., Higgs, P., Hyde, M. and Wiggins, R. (2004) Life course influences on quality of life in early old age, *Social Science and Medicine*, 58: 2171–9.

Blane, D., Montgomery, S. and Berney, L. (1998) Social class differences in lifetime exposure to environmental hazards, *Sociology of Health and Illness*, 20: 532–36.

Blane, D., Netuveli, G. and Bartley, M. (2007) Does quality of life at older ages vary with socio-economic position? *Sociology*, 41: 717–26.

Blane, D., Netuveli, G. and Montgomery, S. (2008) Quality of life, health and physiological status and change at older ages, *Social Science and Medicine*, 66: 1579–87.

Blane, D., Netuveli, G. and Stone, J. (2007) The development of life course epidemiology, *Revue d'Epidemiologie et de Santé Publique*, 55: 31–8.

Breeze, E. and Lang, I. (2008) Physical functioning in a community context, in J. Banks, E. Breeze, C. Lessof and J. Nazroo (eds) *Living in the 21st Century: Older People in England.* London: Institute of Fiscal Studies.

Department of Health (DH) (Committee on the Medical Effects of Air Pollutants) (1998) *Quantification of the Effects of Air Pollution on Health in the United Kingdom.* London: The Stationery Office.

Drever, F. and Whitehead, M. (eds) (1997) *Health Inequalities.* London: The Stationery Office.

Gunnell, D.J., Davey Smith, G., Frankel, S. et al. (1998) Childhood leg length and adult mortality: follow up of the Carnegie (Boyd Orr) Survey of Diet and Health in Pre-war Britain, *Journal of Epidemiology and Community Health*, 52: 142–52.

Gunnell, D.J., Whitley, E., Upton, M.N. et al. (2003) Associations of height, leg length, and lung function with cardiovascular risk factors in the Midspan Family Study, *Journal of Epidemiology and Community Health*, 57: 141–6.

Guralnik, J.M., Butterworth, S., Wadsworth, M.E. and Kuh, D. (2006) Childhood socioeconomic status predicts physical functioning a half century later, *Journals of Gerontology, Series A, Biological Sciences and Medical Sciences*, 61: 694–701.

Hallqvist, J., Lynch, J., Bartley, M., Lange, T. and Blane, D. (2004) Can we disentangle life course processes of accumulation, critical period and social mobility? An analysis of disadvantaged socio-economic positions and myocardial infarction in the Stockholm Heart Epidemiology Program, *Social Science and Medicine*, 58: 1555–62.

Hattersley, L. (1997) Expectation of life by social class, in F. Drever and M. Whitehead (eds) *Health Inequalities*. London: The Stationery Office.

Holland, P., Berney, L., Blane, D. et al. (2000) Life course accumulation of disadvantage, *Social Science and Medicine*, 50: 1285–95.

Khaw, K-T. (1999) Inequalities in health: older people, in G. Gordon, M. Shaw, D. Dorling and G. Davey Smith (eds) *Inequalities in Health: Evidence Presented to Acheson Report*. Bristol: Policy Press.

Kuh, D. and Wadsworth, M. (1989) Parental height: childhood environment and subsequent adult height in a national birth cohort, *International Journal of Epidemiology*, 18: 663–8.

Kuh, D., Richards, M., Hardy, R., Butterworth, S. and Wadsworth, M.E. (2004) Childhood cognitive ability and deaths up until middle age: a post-war birth cohort study, *International Journal of Epidemiology*, 33: 414–15.

Kuh, D.J., Wadsworth, M.E. and Yusuf, E.J. (1994) Burden of disability in a post war birth cohort in the UK, *Journal of Epidemiology and Community Health*, 48: 262–9.

Langenberg, C., Kuh, D., Wadsworth, M.E.J., Brunner, E. and Hardy, R. (2006) Social circumstances and education: life course origins of social inequalities in metabolic risk in a prospective national birth cohort, *American Journal of Public Health*, 96: 2216–21.

Langenberg, C., Shipley, M.J., Batty, G.D. and Marmot, M.G. (2005) Adult socioeconomic position and the association between height and coronary heart disease mortality: findings from 33 years of follow-up in the Whitehall Study, *American Journal of Public Health*, 95: 628–32.

Li, L., Dangour, A.D. and Power, C. (2007) Early life influences on adult leg and trunk length in the 1958 British birth cohort, *Annals of Human Biology*, 19: 836–43.

Mann, S., Wadsworth, M. and Colley, J. (1992) Accumulation of factors influencing respiratory illness in members of a national birth cohort and their offspring, *Journal of Epidemiology and Community Health*, 46: 286–92.

Marmot, M. and Shipley, M. (1996) Do socioeconomic differences in mortality persist after retirement? 25 year follow up of civil servants from the first Whitehall Study, *British Medical Journal*, 313: 1177–80.

Marmot, M., Banks, J., Blundell, R., Lessof, C. and Nazroo, J. (2003) *Health, Wealth and Lifestyles of the Older Population in England: The 2002 English Longitudinal Study of Ageing*. London: Institute of Fiscal Studies.

Maynard, M., Gunnell, D., Abraham, L., Ness, A., Bates, C. and Blane, D. (2006) What influences diet at older ages? Prospective and cross-sectional analyses of the Boyd Orr cohort, *European Journal of Public Health*, 16: 315–23.

Maynard, M., Ness, A., Abraham, L., Blane, D., Bates, C. and Gunnell, D. (2005) Selecting a healthy diet score: lessons from a study of diet and health in early old age (the Boyd Orr cohort), *Public Health Nutrition*, 8: 321–6.

Mitchell, R., Blane, D. and Bartley, M. (2002) Elevated risk of high blood pressure: climate and the inverse housing law, *International Journal of Epidemiology*, 31: 831–8.

Montgomery, S., Berney, L. and Blane, D. (2000) Pre-pubertal growth and blood pressure in early old age, *Archives of Disease in Childhood*, 82: 358–63.

Morris, J.N., Donkin, A., Wonderling, D., Wilkinson, P. and Dowler, E. (2000) A minimum income for healthy living, *Journal of Epidemiology and Community Health*, 54: 885–9.

Morris, J.N., Wilkinson, P., Dangour, A., Deeming, C. and Fletcher, A. (2007) Defining a minimum income for healthy living (MIHL): Older age, England, *International Journal of Epidemiology*, 36: 1300–7.

Nazroo, J., Zaninotto, P. and Gjonca, E. (2008) Mortality and healthy life expectancy, in J. Banks, E. Breeze, C. Lessof and J. Nazroo (eds) *Living in the 21st Century: Older People in England*. London: Institute of Fiscal Studies.

Netuveli, G., Hildon, Z., Montgomery, S., Wiggins, R. and Blane, D. (2005) Need for change in focus from illness to functioning to improve quality of life: evidence from a national survey, *British Medical Journal*, 331: 1382–3.

Netuveli, G., Hildon, Z., Montgomery, S., Wiggins, R. and Blane, D. (2006) Quality of life at older ages: evidence from English Longitudinal Study of Ageing, *Journal of Epidemiology and Community Health*, 60: 357–63.

Netuveli, G., Wiggins, R., Montgomery, S., Hildon, Z. and Blane, D. (2008) Mental health and resilience at older ages: bouncing back after adversity in the British Household Panel Survey, *Journal of Epidemiology and Community Health*, 62: 987–91.

Power, C. and Hertzman, C. (1997) Social and biological pathways linking early life and adult disease, *British Medical Bulletin*, 53: 210–11.

Power, C., Atherton, K., Strachan, D.P. et al. (2007) Life-course influences on health in British adults: effects of socio-economic position in childhood and adulthood, *International Journal of Epidemiology*, 36: 532–9.

Strachan, D.P., Rudnicka, A.R., Power, C. et al. (2007) Lifecourse influences on health among British adults: Effects of region of residence in childhood and adulthood, *International Journal of Epidemiology*, 36: 522–31.

Tabassum, F., Kumari, M., Rumley, A. et al. (2008) Effects of socioeconomic position on inflammatory and hemostatic markers: a life-course analysis in the 1958 British Birth Cohort, *American Journal of Epidemiology*, 167: 1332–41.

Wadsworth, M.E., Hardy, R.J., Paul, A.A., Marshall, S.F. and Cole, T.J. (2002) Leg and trunk length at 43 years in relation to childhood health, diet and family circumstances: evidence from the 1946 national birth cohort, *International Journal of Epidemiology*, 31: 383–90.

Wiggins, R., Higgs, P., Hyde, M. and Blane, D. (2004) Quality of life in the third age: key predictors of the CASP-19 measure, *Aging and Society*, 24: 693–708.

1.3 Geographical inequalities in health over the last century

Danny Dorling and Bethan Thomas

Introduction

A century ago, infant mortality rates in parts of Britain were as high as in the poorest of countries today. Life expectancy similarly and largely as a result was low, but there were still wide variations between different parts of cities, as had been the case throughout the Victorian period. However, it was not until 1921 that statistics were published for areas similar enough to those used today to allow comparisons to be made directly between the present and the past for the whole of Britain.

In this chapter, we review evidence on geographical inequalities in health in Britain from 1921 up to the latest data available: 2006 in England and Wales, and up to the end of 2007 in Scotland. To bring our analysis up to the present, we replicate previous studies with more recent data. To extend it back to 1921, we have expanded past time series back to that year. As part of our analyses, we have calculated for the first time comparable statistics on inequalities in mortality from 1921 up to 2006 across Britain by geographical area.

The central message of our chapter is summarized in Table 1.3.3. Geographical inequalities in mortality ratios under age 65 fell in Britain from 1921 until around 1936. They then rose slightly. In the late 1930s, people living in the worst-off areas were nearly twice as likely to die as those in the best-off. After the Second World War (1939–45), the first published statistics were for the 1950–3 period. These showed that inequality had fallen to a ratio of 1.60. That fall coincided with the 1945–50 Labour government's period of office. The ratio then rose to 1.76 by the end of 1963, before falling again to 1.58, the lowest rate for the entire 1921–2006 period, coincident with another Labour government period of tenure (1964–70). No statistics were available for the period 1973 to 1980 due to cost cutting in the government statistical service by the incoming 1979 government. By the early 1980s, the ratio had risen to 1.70, by the late 1980s to 1.78, by the early 1990s to 1.93 and by the late 1990s to 2.17, the highest ratio for the entire period. Again under another Labour government, the extreme ratio measured for deaths under age 65 fell in the early 2000s, albeit only slightly, to 2.14. However, as the chapter makes clear using other data, when the most recent changes are measured in other ways, they cannot even be described as a slight narrowing of geographical inequalities. What successes there have been in reducing geographical inequalities have been in reducing deaths slightly faster at very young ages in some of the poorest areas, as compared to the reductions of death rates for similarly aged people in the most affluent areas.

It was against the backdrop of widening geographical inequalities in health that New Labour came to office in 1997. Of all the inequalities they had to tackle, they knew what mattered most. The new health secretary, Frank Dobson, spelt it out to the House of Commons. He said 'There are huge inequalities in our society. Poor people are ill more often and die sooner. And that's the greatest inequality of them all – the inequality between the living and the dead' (cited in Warden, 1998: 493). In the late 1990s, the government identified two targets through which to measure the success of their policies in reducing health inequalities. The first focuses on infants for whom information on father's occupation is recorded on the birth certificate and seeks to reduce the gap in death rates in the first year of life between infants born to fathers in working-class occupations ('routine and manual' socio-economic group) and the national average. The second is concerned with the differences in life expectancy found between different areas across the country. Further information on the two targets, and on the socio-economic classification used for the infant mortality target, is provided in Hilary Graham's introductory chapter.

The definitions of both targets were altered over time. But however the targets are measured, in general their progress has been in one direction only: towards greater inequality. Health inequalities have increased year-on-year under New Labour. The only exception to this has been a decline in infant mortality inequalities over the 2004–6 period. Health inequalities reflect inequalities in society in general but are the most obvious and important outcome of the government's failure to tackle inequality locally.[1]

We undertake our review of geographical inequalities in health by beginning with the recent past before looking back at trends over the last century. The next section assesses the evidence on health inequalities from 1996 to 2006 in the two outcomes which form the basis of England's key health inequalities targets: infant mortality and life expectancy. Next, we examine trends in area inequalities from 1990 to 2007 and from 1921 to 2006 as measured by mortality before discussing the role that housing policy could play in tempering area inequalities.

Inequalities in infant mortality and life expectancy from 1996

Figure 1.3.1 focuses on babies whose fathers are in routine and manual occupations, the target group for England's health inequalities target. It shows the percentage by which infant mortality rates among this group of infants have been above average levels in England and Wales for each year between 1996 and 2006 inclusive (the data were taken from DH, 2005, 2006, 2008).[2] If there were no differences between the chances of these babies dying during the first year of life (most in their first few weeks), the bars would have zero height. Note that the scale on the graph starts at the '10' percentage point. That point has not been attained in any of the years between 1996 and 2006. For every 10 babies that die in Britain, 11 die to poorer parents. At times during these years, the inequality has risen to almost 12 babies born to poor parents dying for every 10 that die on average, a 20 per cent higher rate. The statistics were moving towards equality from 1996 to 1998. However, from 1998 to 2004, apart from a 'blip' in 2002, the gap grew relentlessly. It has fallen since 2004 but is still much higher than when the Labour government came to power in 1997.

The widening gap in infant mortality reflects well the growth of the gap between the material living standards of their parents and the average for

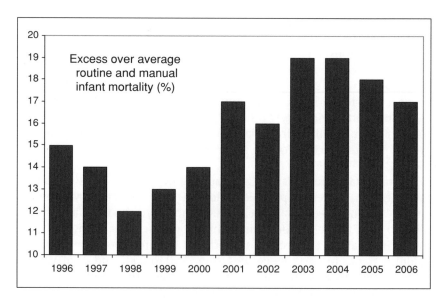

Figure 1.3.1 Infant mortality rates in England and Wales, 1996–2006.

the population. It is important to note that the government's decision to differentiate non-working individuals without children from those with children in the welfare and benefit system has led to many infants being born to new parents who lack the financial support they need during pregnancy. Tax credits, like child benefit and other benefits paid to families with children, can be delivered too slowly to improve the living standards of families for most of these additional children who die so soon after birth. For example, child benefit can only be claimed once the baby is born and registered, and HM Revenue and Customs (2008) 'aim to ... pay you within seven to eight weeks of getting your claim form'. It is interesting to note that the narrowing of the gap in infant mortality since 2004 coincides with the slight fall in material inequalities as measured through income inequalities that occurred about a year prior to then, but which ended in 2005–6 (Institute for Fiscal Studies, 2008).

Figure 1.3.2 shows the difference in life expectancy between the best- and worst-off districts in the UK in the years between 1999 and 2006. The government uses complex measures to calculate inequalities in life expectancy by area, and their preferred measures have changed over time. But the government's figures highlight the same trends of rising inequalities as are seen in infant mortality rates, except with no recent improvement. Figure 1.3.2 illustrates the trend by comparing life expectancies of the populations of the most extreme districts year-on-year. With the largest increases occurring in the most recent years, the figure is hardly good evidence that the continuing widening of the gap is a legacy of a past era of Conservative policies.[3]

The overall life expectancy of a population is a health indicator that responds more slowly to policy interventions than does infant mortality. Part of this widening gap will include the legacy of the different rates at which smoking, for instance, declined by social class in the past. However, the exacerbated sorting of people by social class and ability to pay for housing between areas under New Labour has greatly magnified any such legacy effects (Thomas and Dorling, 2007). Figure 1.3.3 shows the current map of health inequalities, along with one indicating the location of major towns and cities.

Just as the increasing inequalities in infant mortality reflect the increasing material inequalities between poor parents (and most importantly prospective parents) and the rest, so rising inequalities in life expectancy between areas are a mirror of the rising economic inequalities that have emerged so much more clearly than before between different parts of Britain under New Labour. Regional geographical inequalities have risen faster under New Labour than they did under Margaret Thatcher (Dorling et al., 2008). This may not have been the intention, but the effect in terms of relative health inequalities has been devastating.

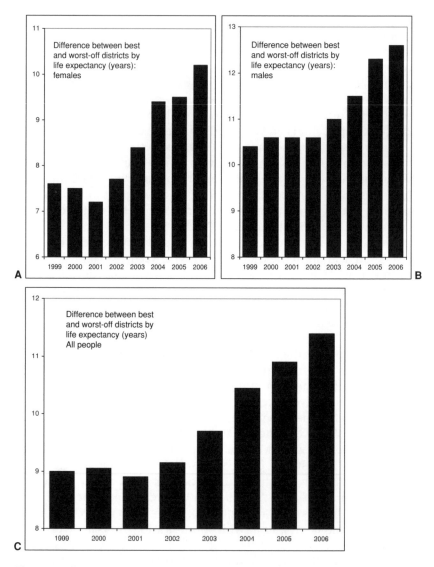

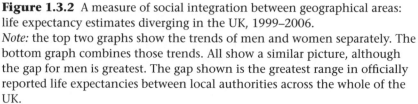

Figure 1.3.2 A measure of social integration between geographical areas: life expectancy estimates diverging in the UK, 1999–2006.
Note: the top two graphs show the trends of men and women separately. The bottom graph combines those trends. All show a similar picture, although the gap for men is greatest. The gap shown is the greatest range in officially reported life expectancies between local authorities across the whole of the UK.

Females   *Males*

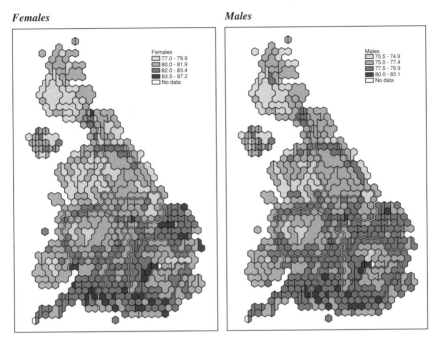

Britain: location of major towns

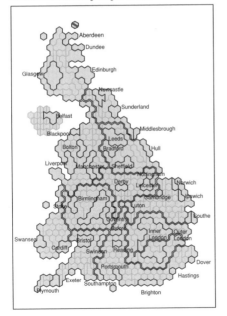

Figure 1.3.3 Life expectancy at birth 2004–6, Britain.
Note: due to their small populations, data are not supplied for the City of London and the Isles of Scilly.

Trends by Standardized Mortality Ratios 1990–2007

For this chapter, we have revised and extended previous work on trends in standardized mortality ratios (SMRs) among the population under the age of 75 (Davey Smith et al., 2002). Revisions were necessary for the 1990s as there were significant revisions to population estimates for the 1990s following the 2001 Census. Because of those revisions to past population at risk estimates, the figures for the early and mid 1990s that we report here are slightly different to those reported earlier. However, the trends are identical.

Standardized mortality ratios (indirect) are the ratios of the observed number of deaths in an area divided by the expected number predicted to occur over a particular time period. The ratios are usually multiplied by 100. The expected number is calculated as the number of deaths that would have been expected to have occurred had the mortality rates by people in the area by age and sex been identical to national average rates. The national average rates we use are those for England and Wales at each time period considered. We recalculated the 1990s SMRs using revised 'Estimating with Confidence' population figures (Norman et al., 2008) for the 1991 Census, aggregated from 1991 census wards to 2001 parliamentary constituencies and interpolating between 1991 and 2001. We calculated SMRs for the parliamentary constituencies of Britain grouped into ten equal (population) sized 'decile' groups when all constituencies were ranked by their experience of poverty as measured around the year 2000. This ranking of poverty is more up to date than we used in our previous work. This again influences the results slightly but the effect of all these changes was, in policy and trend terms, negligible as we illustrate next.

There was in fact minimal change from the previously published results, with the largest change in SMR (due to denominator revision) being 4 percentage points (falling from 109 to 105 for decile 4 in 1990–1). For post-millennium years, we used the mid-year population estimates released by the Office for National Statistics for Census Area Statistics wards for England and Wales and by the Registrar General for Scotland for Datazones; the small area geographical data were aggregated to 2001 parliamentary constituencies. As the 2001 Census and subsequent mid-year population estimates locate students studying away from home at their term-time addresses, we needed to apply a correction factor to relocate students studying away from home to their home constituencies (details can be found in the technical appendix to Shaw et al., 2008).

Mortality data were supplied by the Office for National Statistics (England and Wales) and the General Register Office for Scotland. The data were supplied with the residential postcodes of the deceased which were assigned to the relevant parliamentary constituency. There were a small number of records with no postcodes, and these were not included in the calculations. Such records are generally of visitors to Britain who are not normally resident.[4] Single-year data were combined into two-year groupings. We used the Breadline Britain Index 2000 (Dorling et al., 2007) for ranking parliamentary constituencies into equal-sized population deciles, with the same ranking deciles used for each of the time periods. We used parliamentary constituencies as our basic unit as they are of similar population at risk sizes.

Table 1.3.1 shows the age and sex standardized mortality ratios for death before age 75, the ratio of worst-off to best-off decile, and the Relative Index of Inequality for mortality (RII), for the period 1990–2005. The RII is the relative rate of mortality for the hypothetical poorest compared with the richest in the population. It is calculated here by putting a regression line through a graph of all parliamentary constituencies where they are placed according to their poverty rank on the X axis and their SMR on the Y axis. The RII is the hypothetical worst-off rate divided by the hypothetical best-off and is influenced by all the data points rather than just the extremes. Where the constituency inequality distribution is quite linear, the RII is the same as the decile range. Thus in the 1990–1 period, the RII of 1.61 is identical to the ratio of the worst-off to best-off decile. By 2004–5, the RII was nearly 10 percentage points higher (at 1.91) than the simple ratio (which is 1.8158), indicating that by 2005, considering all constituencies, the gap was wider than if just the extreme deciles were compared.

The RII has risen steadily over the period, but fastest between 1995 and 1997, and slowest between 1999 and 2001. The gap between the SMRs of the most and least deprived deciles widened up to the late 1990s and has remained unchanged since. Put simply, the rot may have almost stopped but there has been no improvement as yet.

Table 1.3.1 shows that, up until the end of 2005, inequalities in mortality by area across Britain were continuing to rise as measured by the relative index of inequality applied to standardised mortality rates (of those dying under age 75). Thus the more complex analysis supports the impression that the simple comparison of life expectancy ranges gives as shown in Figure 1.3.2. We have found through experimentation that inequality change estimates by this method are really only stable when applied to people dying under age 75 if 24 months of data are combined. Thus the columns in Table 1.3.1 all compare pairs of years. This has the added advantage of including two winters so that one 'bad' one does not have too much influence. Similarly, tainted heroin, a scare over immunization

Table 1.3.1 Age and sex standardized SMRs (0–74) according to decile of poverty and the relative index of inequality, Britain, 1990–2006

SMR 0–74	1990–1	1992–3	1994–5	1996–7	1998–9	2000–1	2002–3	2004–5	2005–6
Decile 1	129	132	135	137	138	139	138	138	138
Decile 2	116	118	118	120	121	119	121	121	121
Decile 3	113	115	114	115	115	116	117	117	116
Decile 4	105	107	106	108	109	109	107	108	108
Decile 5	103	102	102	101	103	103	103	103	104
Decile 6	96	94	95	94	95	95	96	95	96
Decile 7	91	90	90	90	89	90	90	90	90
Decile 8	86	86	85	85	84	84	85	86	85
Decile 9	85	83	83	82	81	81	81	81	80
Decile 10	80	79	79	78	77	76	76	76	76
Ratio	1.61	1.67	1.71	1.76	1.79	1.83	1.82	1.82	1.82
RII	1.61	1.67	1.71	1.81	1.86	1.86	1.90	1.91	1.89

Note: the final column is not a direct continuation of the series but the latest-available two years' data.

for influenza, suicides falling or rising in response to particular events, has less of an impact over a two-year time period.

We do not yet have access to mortality data for 2007 for England and Wales and so, in the interim, we have calculated a final column for the years 2005–6. This produces the intriguing possibility that there has been a reduction in the relative index of inequality. Note that the overall range between deciles remains at 1.82 since 2001 with no change evident in the most recent time period (2005–6). This equates to 82 per cent more people in the worst-off decile dying each year under age 75 than in the best-off having allowed for age and sex differences. It is possible that our population denominators are becoming biased with distance from the 2001 Census so we are cautious about placing too much weight on this result. However, if it was confirmed when data for 2007 become available, then it may become possible to claim, finally, that the gap between the health of areas in Britain had stopped widening by 2007.

We do currently have access to mortality data for Scotland for the year 2007. As standardized mortality rates in Scottish constituencies are the highest in Britain, it is worth looking at trends there to try to gain an impression of whether the gap might be beginning to close. Table 1.3.2 shows the absolute numbers of people who died, each year 2004 to 2007, in each of the ten Scottish constituencies with the highest mortality ratios in recent years. These are the 2007 Scottish parliamentary constituencies,

Table 1.3.2 The numbers of deaths in the ten Scottish constituencies with the worst standardized mortality ratios (SMRs) in 2006

Constituency	Number of deaths			
	2004	2005	2006	2007
Airdrie and Shotts	406	392	433	448
Glasgow Anniesland	317	340	322	324
Glasgow Baillieston	378	327	328	346
Glasgow Cathcart	267	194	232	283
Glasgow Govan	316	364	370	330
Glasgow Maryhill	417	328	321	368
Glasgow Pollok	443	387	383	397
Glasgow Shettleston	461	364	402	393
Glasgow Springburn	528	509	500	472
Paisley North	350	403	411	348
Total	3,883	3,608	3,702	3,709

that is those used to elect Members of the Scottish Parliament (the same as 2001 Westminster parliamentary constituencies; new Scottish constituencies for the Westminster parliament were created for 2005 but we do not use those here).

Between 2006 and 2007, in only 4 of the 10 Scottish parliamentary constituencies do the number of these deaths fall. The total number of deaths remains lower in 2007 than it was in 2004, but there is still no clear sign here of improvements in areas with the worst health profile. These are actual counts of people who have died, not age- and sex-adjusted figures, as population estimates by age and sex for 2007 are not yet available.

Trends by standardized mortality ratio 1921–2006

In previous work, we described standardized mortality ratios for the period 1950 to 1992 by decile areas of Britain for deaths under age 65 (Shaw et al., 1998). Due to limitations of the data for the 1950s to 1970s, these statistics used only five age bands (age 0, 1–4, 5–14, 15–44 and 45–64) for men and women, and were of areas amalgamated from the 1974 local authorities and sorted at each time period by SMR before being grouped by each population decile.

Table 1.3.3 shows these statistics, with those for the 1990–2 period replaced by revised data, and 1993–2006 and 1921–39 data added. The penultimate row of the table is the ratio of worst-off to best-off decile.

Table 1.3.3 Standardized mortality ratio 0–64 (1921–2006)

Decile	1921–5	1926–30	1931–5	1936–9	1950–3	1959–63	1969–73	1981–5	1986–9	1990–2	1993–5	1996–7	1999–2001	2002–4	2004–6
1	141.1	136.7	134.9	136.3	131.0	135.5	131.2	135.0	139.2	144.3	148.9	152.6	151.3	150.4	149.1
2	123.9	121.7	119.7	119.6	118.1	123.0	115.6	118.6	120.9	122.1	121.7	123.0	123.9	124.1	123.4
3	114.0	111.8	111.7	111.7	112.1	116.5	112.0	114.2	113.9	112.8	113.5	114.9	115.6	115.2	116.3
4	107.8	107.3	105.9	106.5	107.0	110.7	108.1	109.8	106.9	106.8	106.8	109.0	108.0	108.0	108.7
5	102.5	102.8	102.2	102.8	102.5	104.5	103.0	102.1	102.2	99.6	98.4	98.3	99.7	100.2	100.8
6	95.6	97.0	97.5	96.9	98.6	97.4	96.9	95.7	95.6	93.7	93.7	94.2	94.7	94.7	95.5
7	89.7	89.9	90.3	90.3	93.1	90.9	91.8	91.6	91.9	90.7	90.6	90.7	90.1	90.7	89.7
8	83.9	82.9	83.8	84.6	88.7	87.6	88.9	89.3	89.1	86.0	85.4	85.1	83.0	82.3	82.8
9	77.3	79.0	80.6	80.3	85.7	83.1	87.0	84.3	83.0	79.6	78.7	76.8	77.2	76.7	76.0
10	70.0	74.7	74.0	70.9	81.8	77.1	83.0	79.2	78.1	74.6	72.3	70.7	69.7	70.2	69.7
Ratio	2.02	1.83	1.82	1.92	1.60	1.76	1.58	1.70	1.78	1.93	2.06	2.16	2.17	2.14	2.14
RII	2.64	2.41	2.33	2.41	1.96	2.25	1.92	2.12	2.22	2.49	2.64	2.80	2.85	2.83	2.84

Notes:

1. The time periods vary due to data limitations; in particular, there is a large gap between 1939 and 1950.
2. For 1990 (included in 1990–2), 1991 population figures were used. For 2006 (included in 2004–6), 2005 mid-year estimates (the latest available at small area geography) were used.
3. The final column does not follow on but overlaps; it is the latest three years for which mortality data were available for all of Britain.

In the period 1921 to 1925, the worst-off tenth of the population by area had an age-sex standardized mortality rate below age 65 that was 41 per cent higher than the national average of the time. The best-off tenth had a rate which was 70 per cent of the national average. The ratio of worst-off to best-off tenth was 141/70 = 2.02. Thus in any given year, a person aged under 65 was twice as likely to die if they lived in the worst-off areas rather than in the best-off.

The ratio of 2.02 in the 1920s had fallen slightly by the end of the 1930s to 1.92. It then fell sharply to 1953, then rose in the 1950s to 1963 (under a Conservative government), before falling from 1964 through to 1973. At some point in the late 1970s, the tide turned and the gap steadily widened. The last row of the table shows the RII from 1921 to 2006. The story told using the Relative Index of Inequality is identical in terms of the timings of the improvements of these trends being coincident with post-war Labour governments and dramatic increases in mortality inequalities under the 1979–96 Conservative government carrying on into the first two years of the New Labour government.

The data for the most recent period enables us to measure changes in the RII since 2001. Comparing 2002–4 with 2004–6, health inequalities between areas for deaths under age 65 have increased again, albeit by a single percentage point from 2.83 to 2.84, with the latter figure being just below the 1991–2000 maxima of 2.85.

Discussion

Clearly, by 2007, relative health inequalities in Britain had reached levels greater than the early 1920s. Inequalities may be about to fall, although if they do fall it would need to be in poor parts of England that the mortality falls begin. We would expect London to lead the way as the poorest London boroughs have benefited from high rates of immigration (and almost all immigrants tend to be healthier than those they join). The monitoring of these trends is important, but what matters most is reducing the inequalities. To reduce health inequalities between areas requires reducing general inequalities between areas so that people do not try disproportionately to leave places such as the ten listed in Table 1.3.2, when they are able. It also requires policies that allow people who might have poorer health and lower financial resources to live in more affluent areas. A 'right to sell' your house to the council and become a tenant would be one mechanism that could be introduced to achieve this.

If we were to suggest one policy that would help achieve this, it would be to extend the scheme allowing and assisting social landlords to purchase homes at auction and those being offered for private sale on the market for which, in late 2007 and throughout 2008 at least, there were no buyers. It would need central funding given that one of the banks that went 'bust' in 2008, Bradford and Bingley, was one of the largest funders of housing associations. It would result in the achievement of numerous government goals on social mixing, reducing local inequalities, stabilizing the housing market and so on. In few other circumstances would it be popular among home owners than during the recession that began in late summer 2007. And it could help reduce the massive disappointment of the 60,000 people now registered, say, on Sheffield's housing waiting list, or the estimated 4 million people registered nationally for a council or housing association home (Local Government Association, 2008). Area health inequalities in places like Sheffield are stark because housing inequalities are so stark. If there were much more social housing in those parts of cities, like Sheffield, that had the least social housing to begin with, it is hard to see how health inequalities within Sheffield would not fall.

Social inequalities in Britain as a whole have been rising in recent decades (Dorling et al., 2008) and this has led to a spatial polarization of the population by poverty and wealth and consequently health. If social inequalities continue to rise, housing is likely to be distributed more and more inequitably. It is much more how we distribute wealth and opportunity within the country that determines how well people are housed than how many people chose to live in each place, not to leave, are not so desperate to move in, and so on (Dorling, 2009).

If we wish to see health inequalities fall between areas, we need to match type of housing supply to need. In some areas, high proportions of one/two-bed flats have been built but people want houses with gardens. In many affluent parts of London, there are homes which are empty for much for the week because the occupants live elsewhere. Many homes in and around London and in other particular cities are not occupied at weekends. There has been an explosion in the ownership of second homes and this exacerbates area inequalities (National Housing and Planning Advice Unit, 2008). This under-use of housing is also often in close proximity to areas where children are often living below the official bedroom standard.

The social divisions between people have changed more obviously in recent years when people are sorted by address rather than occupation; this suggests slow and steady increases in social immobility over time (Dorling et al., 2007). The address you are born in matters more now than it did in the 1940s, 1950s, 1960s and 1970s for your chances of dying young, being poor or wealthy and so on. Wealth inequalities also matter more than income inequalities now as compared to the recent past (Dorling, 2008). Inequalities in wealth, and particularly in housing wealth, have, like health inequalities, risen over time. We have noted elsewhere that in Britain

> in the best off tenth of areas the housing wealth per child has increased by 20 times more than that of the lowest decile since

1993. The children of Great Britain are clearly becoming quickly more differentiated through the relative wealth of their families. Much is written about rising student debt and similar problems. Very little is said about the increase, in just ten years, of £61,842 per child in the housing wealth of families with children living where prices have risen the most in ten years. At current prices, if the housing wealth of the best tenth of families by area is shared out amongst their children that housing wealth was £82,490 per child by the end of 2003. As house prices rise over the medium and long term (if not the short term) the real wealth gap will be much greater in future.

(Thomas and Dorling, 2004: 5)

The rapid onset of national and global recession in 2008 has dented political and public faith in markets: the assumption that the choices of those with most money are the 'best choices' has taken a hit. In key issues such as housing, education and health, governments will need to do more with less in the future. This will require an increase in efficiency, and it is going to be very hard for those brought up under orthodox economic thinking to cope with this change. However, such a change in thinking at the centre offers the chance to enable any halt in the decade-on-decade widening of area health inequalities to be translated into a sustained narrowing in health inequalities. In the 1950s and 1960s, there were no areas of Britain where people were a quarter more likely than average to die young simply due to where they lived.

Conclusion

In this chapter, our major focus has been on changes over time in relative health inequalities between areas in Britain from 1921 to 2006. We began by discussing England's two key targets for health inequalities: the area-based life expectancy target and the infant mortality target designed to level up life chances for infants in poorer families. We have discussed how there has been a slow-down in the rise in inequalities in health, but no actual fall, as yet, in those inequalities. Inequalities in mortality rates between areas of Britain were, by the end of 2001, at their highest for the entire period 1921–2006.

Life expectancy in the wealthy parts of London – in Kensington and Chelsea – have in recent years been recorded as rising by slightly more than a year each year. In the poorest districts, rates have been hardly rising at all. Current rates of growth in area health inequalities are unsustainable. Rises of a year every year in life expectancy, if sustained, result in immortality. That alone tells us that we have been living through very strange times. Of course, such rises are unsustainable because immortality is not possible: life expectancy in areas where it was already high cannot carry on rising as quickly. Similarly, there are levels below which infant mortality cannot fall (probably of around 1 infant dying per 1000 born). Partly because of this, we should expect inequalities in infant health to improve in the future. The fact that we are not immortal should not be a comfort to those in the New Labour government who hope to welcome the turning of the trend in these graphs as proof that their policies have finally worked. When compared to the stated aims of New Labour when it came to power in 1997, what has been allowed to occur over the last ten years has been an abject failure. Ensuring economic circumstances that make the lives of the rich and poor less different – essentially ensuring that there are fewer who are disproportionately rich and fewer who are disproportionately poor – will have similar effects in both the immediate and longer term. There is no efficient alternative to increasing economic equality if the government's aim is a motivated, well-educated and healthy population.

Governments have a traditional trick of suggesting that, at any moment now, things are going to get better, the data are just a little bit old, signs of a turnaround are in the air, we are spending so much, are so committed, and so on. Improving disadvantaged areas has been a government priority for improving health; clearly not enough of a priority. A government that proposes to narrow the inequalities gap by helping people to make 'healthier choices' in their daily lives is likely to be one which is out of touch with the realities of life for the most disadvantaged. Health inequalities in Britain did not occur, increase and persist because people 'chose' not to be healthy and because people 'chose' poverty.

At some point soon, calculations will be made of the number of babies that would have lived to see their first birthday, the number of women who would not have seen their children die before them and the number of men who would have made it to 65 years had New Labour achieved its ambitions to reduce inequalities in health in the period May 1997 to May 2007. All these infants and children and adults have now died. By far the greatest proportion will be those that voted Labour in 1997, or whose parents and grandparents had voted Labour in both that year and were the basis of that party's success in the past. Perhaps every Labour MP and Minister needs this list (Dorling, 1998)[5] to help them understand who among those they represented from 1997 are no longer here as a result of this policy failure. If we do not learn that what has been achieved since 1997 is not enough – for so many people – then there is little point in counting the dead.

In 1936, Britain was in the depths of economic recession. Very few people would have imagined that within 14 years mortality rates between areas would be at their most equal. In 2006, Britain was approaching the end of the longest-ever economic boom in its recorded history. But it was living with levels of geographical inequalities in health that were higher than those 1936 levels – and which were still rising slightly when counted in some ways. Anyone expressing the hope that within 14 years – by 2020 – mortality rate ratios between areas could be reduced to levels last seen in the 1950s would sound as utopian as their equivalents in 1936. Except, of course, in 1936 nobody knew of any of these trends.

Notes

1. There is, of course, a far greater body count that will dominate the history of New Labour (see McPherson, 2005). As McPherson notes, 'counting the dead is intrinsic to civilised society. Understanding the causes of death is a core public health responsibility' (2005:550).
2. Note that infant mortality figures are for England and Wales only; figures are for the three-year period ending December of the date shown.
3. It was of course the Conservative governments of 1979–97 that saw and helped the gap widen from historically low levels of inequality experienced in the 1950s, 1960s and early 1970s.
4. Similarly, there were a small number of records with no cause of death given. As the ages of the deceased in these records ranged from the full age range in some years' data, to all the ages being zero in other years, these records too were discarded from the analysis.
5. The list of potential victims of policy failure was drawn up shortly after the 1997 election victory. Table 5 in Dorling (1998) listed the number of voters who would continue to die young from 1997 onwards, by their MPs, in the worse-off areas, were inequalities to remain so high. Many of those Labour MPs whose constituents have suffered most due to the failure to narrow inequalities have had the power to change policy. Past and current Ministers include Hazel Blears who loses over 100 potential voters a year due to the continuation of such inequalities: 1000 excess young deaths in her constituency since she first contended her Salford seat. There are 750 fewer folk to vote for John Reid now where he has been MP since 1997; 640 fewer for Jack Straw; 590 less for Harriet Harman; and 360 less in the Dunfermline East constituency of Gordon Brown. These deaths are all due to the continued extent of inequalities in life chances in the UK. These figures all represent people who have died before they reached age 65 because rates in their area remain so much in excess of the national average. When these figures were first calculated, they were the hypothetical deaths that would result from policy failure. Now they are gravestones in cemeteries and plaques in crematoria: memorials to lives that need not have ended so soon. For

a few MPs, enough of their constituents have died both prematurely and unnecessarily since 1997 to have been able to fill the House of Commons from their constituency's toll alone. It may well have been worse had another party won power in 1997, but for so many it could have been so much better.

Acknowledgements

We would like to thank the Rowntree Foundation, the British Academy and the Leverhulme Trust for funding Danny Dorling and John Pritchard for his work on the pre-war data.

References

Davey Smith, G., Dorling, D., Mitchell, R. and Shaw, M. (2002) Health inequalities in Britain: continuing increases up to the end of the 20th century, *Journal of Epidemiology and Community Health*, 56: 434–5.

Department of Health (DH) (2005) *Tackling Health Inequalities: Status Report on the Programme for Action*. London: DH.

Department of Health (DH) (2006) *Tackling Health Inequalities: 2003–05 Data Update for the National 2010 PSA Targe*. London: DH.

Department of Health (DH) (2008) *Tackling Health Inequalities: 2007 Status Report on the Programme for Action*. London: DH.

Dorling, D. (1998) Whose voters suffer if inequalities in health remain? *Journal of Contemporary Health*, 7: 50–4.

Dorling, D. (2008) Cash and the not so classless society, *Fabian Review*, 120: 2.

Dorling, D. (2009) *Migration: A Long-run Perspective*. London: Institute of Public Policy Research.

Dorling, D., Mitchell, R., Orford, S. and Shaw, M. (2005) Inequalities and Christmas yet to come, *British Medical Journal*, 331: 1409.

Dorling, D., Rigby, J., Wheeler, B., Ballas, D. et al. (2007) *Poverty, Wealth and Place in Britain, 1968 to 2005*. Bristol: Policy Press.

Dorling, D., Vickers, D., Thomas, B., Pritchard, J. and Ballas, D. (2008) *Britain on the Move: The Change in Our Neighbourhood Today*, Report commissioned by BBC regions and nations. Available at: www.sasi.group.sheff.ac.UK/research/changingUK.html

HM Revenue and Customs (2008) *When to Expect Your First Child Benefit Payment*. Available at www.hmrc.gov.uk/childbenefit/expect-first-child.htm.

Institute for Fiscal Studies (IFS) (2008) *Racing Away? Income Inequality and the Evolution of High Incomes*. London: IFS.

Local Government Association (LGA) (2008) *Councils and the Housing Crisis*. London: LGA.

McPherson, K. (2005) Counting the dead in Iraq, *British Medical Journal*, 330: 550–1.

National Housing and Planning Advice Unit (2008) *Rapid Evidence Assessment of the Research Literature on the Purchase and Use of Second Homes*. Fareham: National Housing and Planning Advice Unit.

Norman, P., Simpson, L. and Sabater, A. (2008) Estimating with confidence and hindsight: new UK small area population estimates for 1991, *Population, Space and Place*, 14: 449–72.

Office for National Statistics (ONS) (2006) *Life Expectancy at Age 65 Continues to Rise*. Press release 21 November, London: ONS.

Shaw, M., Dorling, D. and Brimblecombe, N. (1998) Changing the map: health in Britain 1951–91, *Sociology of Health and Illness*, 20: 694–709.

Shaw, M., Thomas, B., Davey Smith, G. and Dorling, D. (2008) *The Grim Reaper's Road Map: An Atlas of Mortality in Britain*. Bristol: Policy Press.

Thomas, B. and Dorling, D. (2004) *Know Your Place: Housing Wealth and Inequality in Great Britain 1980–2003 and Beyond*. London: Shelter.

Thomas, B. and Dorling D. (2007) *Identity in Britain: A Cradle-to-grave Atlas*. Bristol: Policy Press.

Warden, J. (1998) Britain's new health policy recognises poverty as major cause of illness, *British Medical Journal*, 316: 493.

1.4 Neighbourhood influences on health

Sally Macintyre and Anne Ellaway

Introduction

Information about the interrelationship between residential neighbourhoods, social advantage or disadvantage, and disease or health, has been available for many centuries. A rather elegant illustration is given in Edwin Chadwick's *Sanitary Conditions of the Labouring Poor in Great Britain* (1842), which collated information from a number of sources including reports sent in by Medical Officers of Health in a wide range of areas in the first part of the 19th century. Chadwick used maps relating mortality to the social composition of different areas, and in his report he noted that

> to obtain the means of judging of the references to the localities in the sanitary returns from Aberdeen, the reporters were requested to mark on a map the places where the disease fell, and to distinguish with a deeper tint those places on which it fell with the greatest intensity. They were also requested to distinguish by different colours the streets inhabited by the higher, middle and lower classes of society. They returned a map so marked as to disease, but stated that it had been thought unnecessary to distinguish the streets inhabited by the different orders of society, as that was done with sufficient accuracy by the different tints representing the degrees of the prevalence of fever.
>
> (quoted in Flinn, 1965: 225–6)

This confirms accounts provided by other public health investigators into urban health in the 17th, 18th and early 19th centuries, which showed close correlations between the social composition of neighbourhoods and their death rates (for example, John Graunt's *Natural and Political Observations upon the Bills of Mortality* published in 1662, and Villerme's work on Parisian arrondissements in 1817–21; Macintyre and Ellaway, 2003).

Such observations have continued to be made in the 20th and 21st centuries, and major enquiries into inequalities in health such as the Black report (Black et al., 1980) and the Acheson report (Acheson, 1998) have noted the existence of geographical as well as socio-economic inequalities in health.

Geographical inequalities can be observed at a number of levels, for example between countries, between regions or towns within countries and between small areas within towns or urban areas. In this chapter we focus on urban neighbourhoods, both because this is a spatial scale on which there is a considerable body of recent research, and because this is one which policymakers use both for routine data gathering and monitoring – for example, the UK's neighbourhood statistics (ONS, 2008) and Scotland's indices of multiple deprivation (Scottish Executive, 2004) – and for area-based initiatives.

There are definitional issues around the concept of neighbourhoods both within sociology and urban geography (Galster, 2001). However, for the purposes of this chapter, we are referring to relatively small geographical areas around where people live, and which researchers and policymakers use for analysis and planning purposes, and which residents use for immediate access for activities of daily living (Kearns and Parkinson, 2001).

We do not assume that neighbourhoods have fixed boundaries that are identical for all residents, or that residents' lives are completely contained within their residential neighbourhood. The amount of time people spend in their residential neighbourhood, and the distances people may range for what type of activities, may differ both by their own circumstances and the characteristics of the area, as may their sense of identity and social relations within their local area. In a study of neighbourhood differences in Glasgow, for example, we found that there were differences between neighbourhoods in whether certain activities (such as food shopping, dog walking, doing sport) were done locally or not, even when controlling for age, gender and social class; these differences were related to features of local opportunity structures and the built and natural environment (Macintyre and Ellaway, 1998).

In this chapter, we describe the extent to which neighbourhoods appear to influence health, over and above the characteristics of their residents; some frameworks which seek to explain the ways in which neighbourhoods might influence health; how features of neighbourhoods might be associated with specific health behaviours and health outcomes; how neighbourhoods might fit into models of the generation and maintenance of health inequalities; and how associations between neighbourhoods and health might vary by age, gender, broader national context and historical period. We conclude by noting some gaps in the research literature, and implications for policy.

Measurement and characterization of neighbourhoods

There are a number of ways in which neighbourhoods are measured and characterized. Deprivation indices, for example, typically draw on census data (e.g. proportion of adults who are unemployed or the proportion of dwellings which are overcrowded) and other official statistics (e.g. the proportion of adults in receipt of benefits such as income support and the proportion without educational qualifications) to capture multiple disadvantage at the small area level. This information is used to construct a score which can be applied to small areas at a variety of spatial scales to inform the planning and targeting of services and resources. The spatial scales used in the UK include Super Output Areas (SOAs) which are small areas specifically introduced to improve the reporting and comparison of local statistics; within England and Wales, there is a Lower Layer (minimum population 1000) and a Middle Layer (minimum population 5000). These SOA layers are of consistent size across the country and are not subjected to regular boundary change. In Northern Ireland, there is a single layer of SOAs with minimum population 1300. The Scottish equivalents of SOAs are 'data zones' (minimum population 500) and 'intermediate zones' (minimum population 2500). Areas can also be ranked according to their degree of affluence or deprivation relative to other areas across a city or country.

Are neighbourhoods associated with health and health inequalities?

In the 1990s, there was debate about whether observed neighbourhood differences in health were a result of composition (the characteristics, such as the social class, of residents) or whether they were a result of context (the characteristics, such as the built or social environment, of the place). Most commentators now accept that individual characteristics such as gender or social class are the main predictors of health and health behaviours, but that there is a small independent effect of area characteristics (Pickett and Pearl, 2001; Riva et al., 2007). This has been shown for a wide range of health outcomes, including total mortality, coronary heart disease (CHD) mortality, CHD prevalence and depression, and for health-related behaviours like diet, physical activity, smoking and alcohol consumption. One recent systematic review of multi-level studies concluded that 10 per cent of the variation in health outcomes among children and adolescents was explained by neighbourhood determinants (Sellstrom and Bremberg, 2006).

The extent to which neighbourhood matters for health outcomes (after taking individual characteristics into account) varies by country context. For example, studies of low birthweight have found that women in disadvantaged US neighbourhoods had a 10–20 per cent increased risk of giving birth to an infant with low weight or intra-uterine growth retardation (O'Campo et al., 1997). UK studies have found 10–12 per cent increased risk (Spencer et al., 1999; Aveyard et al., 2002) whereas Nordic countries such as Sweden find only minor differences (less than 1%) between neighbourhoods (Sellstrom et al., 2007) despite concentrations of low income, unemployment and exposure to violence. The ways in which welfare institutions and benefits are provided and resourced in Sweden might buffer against stressful neighbourhood conditions (Sellstrom et al., 2007).

Most commentators also now accept that a rigid distinction between composition and context is difficult and may be theoretically unsound, since over time people create places, and places create people (for example, Macintyre et al., 2002; Barnard et al., 2007). However, even though, as some have argued, it may be theoretically and methodologically impossible completely to separate compositional from contextual effects, for the purposes of policy making, and of furthering our understanding of the processes which generate and maintain inequalities in health, it is still useful to think about how neighbourhoods might influence the health and health behaviours of their residents. An important element of many government strategies to reduce inequalities in health has been to focus on area-based initiatives, and at a high level of policy formation it is important to know whether it is more cost-effective to concentrate on people or places, or how to combine a place-based and people-based approach (Macintyre, 2007).

Why would neighbourhoods be associated with health and health inequalities?

Neighbourhood of residence may be associated with health and the ability to lead a healthy life, and contribute to health inequalities, in a variety of ways. For example, concerns are increasing over the rising levels of obesity and a number of studies have shown that people living in deprived areas are more likely to be overweight or obese, even after taking other known correlates of obesity into account such as age or socio-economic status (SES) (Ellaway et al., 1997; Ross et al., 2007). The mechanisms through which neighbourhood might influence obesity include the availability of shops nearby selling healthy foods at affordable prices and the presence of local facilities and amenities which might encourage physical activity (e.g. swimming pools, sports centres, parks). However, an area may be well equipped with these amenities but if people feel unsafe moving around their neighbourhood, if public transport is poor or if they feel that the facilities are 'not for them' they might be deterred from using facilities. Similarly, if the prevailing norm locally is for people to be overweight or obese, then there may less motivation for individuals to lose weight. Health inequalities between more affluent and deprived areas may be further widened if deprived areas consistently lack access to local health-promoting opportunities or perceptions of safety are lower and this is combined with personal disadvantage such as low income or unemployment.

We have previously suggested the framework in Box 1.4.1 for explaining and analysing potential pathways by which neighbourhoods might influence health (Macintyre et al., 1993):

Box 1.4.1:   Potential pathways by which neighbourhoods might influence health

1. Physical features of the environment shared by all residents in a locality (for example, air and water quality);
2. Availability of healthy environments at home, work and play (for example, decent housing, secure and non-hazardous employment, safe play areas for children);
3. Services provided to support people in their daily lives (for example, education, transport, street cleaning and lighting, and policing);
4. The socio-cultural features of a locality (for example, its political, economic, ethnic and religious history, the degree of community integration);
5. The reputation of an area (for example, how the area is perceived by residents, service or amenity planners, and investors)

Source: adapted from Macintyre et al. (1993).

Other similar frameworks have been put forward. For example Ellen et al. (2001) suggest four mechanisms for neighbourhood influences on health: (1) neighbourhood institutions and resources such as the food environment; (2) stressors in the physical environment such as polluting factories or poor-quality housing; (3) stressors in the social environment such as crime, victimization or noise; and (4) neighbourhood-based networks and norms.

We have suggested that a useful starting point is to think about what human beings need to lead a healthy life, and how these needs may be met at a neighbourhood or larger spatial scale (Macintyre et al., 2002).

These needs include the essentials of life such as air, water, food, shelter, security, and hygiene; and extend through education, transport, work, income, information and communication, and health care, through to more spiritual and social dimensions such as family life, social relations, religious expression, and play. The underlying hypothesis of much work on neighbourhoods and health is that the means for meeting these needs are systematically structured and distributed both by socio-economic status and type of area of residence, in ways which create observed inequalities. In this chapter, given space constraints, we will concentrate on what is known about how the means of meeting such basic human needs are differentially distributed, focusing in particular on the distribution of resources and amenities.

The distribution of resources and amenities

Two major but somewhat separate literatures suggest that poorer places may pose more health risks because of the ways in which health-promoting and health-damaging resources are distributed. The 'inverse care law' suggests that

> the availability of good medical care tends to vary inversely with the need for it in the population served. This inverse care law operates more completely where medical care is most exposed to market forces, less so where such exposure is reduced.
>
> (Tudor Hart, 1971: 405)

We and others have suggested that this is part of a more general pattern, which we call deprivation amplification, by which a range of resources and facilities which might promote health are less common in poorer areas (Macintyre et al., 1993). A similar but converse idea is encapsulated in the notion of environmental injustice, which suggests that environmental threats to health (e.g. waste-disposal sites, air pollution, toxic factory fumes) are more likely to be located in poorer areas (Hofrichter, 1993). The concepts of deprivation amplification and environmental injustice have proved attractive to many social inequalities theorists and policymakers, because they avoid the victim-blaming approach of assuming that health is poor in certain areas because people living there behave badly, or that unhealthy people drift or migrate into certain types of area. They have clear policy and causal implications, for example that diet, nutrition, and levels of obesity are worse in poor areas because they are food deserts and the inhabitants are deprived of the opportunity to access affordable nutritious food. The perceived solutions are then supply-side ones, for example using planning regulations to ensure equitable provision of healthy food or sports facilities.

However, these solutions need to take account of empirical evidence about the distribution and use of resources, or the role of agency, demand, and culture in shaping both what is in a neighbourhood, and how it is used. Much of the recent literature showing deprivation amplification comes from the USA. For example in the USA, higher SES areas have more physical fitness facilities, membership sports and recreation clubs, dance facilities and public golf courses; such facilities were least likely to be present in areas with higher proportions of African-American, Hispanic or other ethnic minority backgrounds (Powell et al., 2006). Similarly, low SES and predominantly black areas lack services such as supermarkets (for example, see Zenk et al., 2005). However, these patterns are not necessarily observed elsewhere. In Australia, lower SES areas in Perth had better access to sports/recreation centres, gyms and swimming pools, while higher SES areas had better access to golf courses and the beach (Giles-Corti and Donovan, 2002); in Melbourne there were no differences in the provision of free access, restricted access or sporting/recreation open spaces by neighbourhood SES (Ball et al., 2006); and there were minimal socio-economic differences in food shopping infrastructure in Brisbane (Winkler et al., 2006). A Dutch study observed no differences by neighbourhood SES in proximity to sports facilities, and closer proximity to food shops with increasing socio-economic disadvantage (van Lenthe et al., 2005). In New Zealand, travel distances to supermarkets are less in more deprived areas (Pearce et al., 2007). Some potentially health-promoting resources, such as children's playgrounds, have consistently been found to be more prevalent in poorer areas even in the USA (see, for example, Cradock et al., 2005).

In the light of these rather differing findings, two groups have recently taken a more systematic approach to examining the geographic distribution of a wide range of health resources. A very comprehensive study of the whole of New Zealand found that for 15 out of 16 measures of community resources, access was clearly better in more deprived neighbourhoods (the only resource which was closer to more affluent neighbourhoods being the beach) (Pearce et al., 2007). Taking a slightly different approach, we tried to operationalize our model of resources needed to meet basic human needs on the scale of a single city, and sought information on the location of as wide a range of resources as possible by neighbourhood deprivation in Glasgow (Macintyre et al., 2008a). We found that some resources were more prevalent in, or closer to, deprived neighbourhoods; others more prevalent in, and closer to, more affluent neighbourhoods; and others showed no relationship to neighbourhood deprivation. A summary of our findings is shown in Box 1.4.2. We found that historical, economic and geographical explanations of this patterning were more useful than simple socio-economic deprivation ones; for example, many resources such

Box 1.4.2: Distribution of amenities by socio-economic deprivation in Glasgow, 2005–6

More/closer to poor areas	*More/closer to rich areas*	*Unrelated to deprivation*
LEA nurseries	LEA secondary schools	Private nurseries
LEA primary schools	Private schools	General practices
Fire stations	Banks	Dental practices
Police stations	Building societies	Opthalmic practices
Pharmacies	Museums/art galleries	Pawnbrokers
Credit unions	Cinemas	Supermarkets
Post offices	Tourist attractions	Fast food chains
Bingo halls	Railway stations	Public libraries
Public swimming pools	Subway stations	Golf courses
Public sports centres	Tennis courts	Parks
Outdoor play areas	Bowling greens	
Vacant and derelict land	Private health clubs	
	Private swimming pools	
	FE colleges	
	A & E hospitals	
	Waste disposal/recycling sites	

Source: adapted from Macintyre et al. (2008a), Table 1.

as banks, ATMs, and cafes are located close to the central business district and major service or shopping areas where there is a lot of passing trade; the railway system was built in the 19th century and middle-class housing developed around stations which provided easy access to the city centre; bingo halls are created in areas where there is likely to be a demand for them; the peripheral council housing estates which were built to house people cleared from the slums after the Second World War were built on cheap empty land, and priority was given to housing rather than community resources; Credit Unions developed in areas with a high proportion of poor people without bank accounts.

Thus, we and others have increasingly found that there is no universal and straightforward picture in which health-promoting resources are more likely to be found in less deprived neighbourhoods, and health-damaging ones in more deprived neighbourhoods; rather, the spatial distribution of resources by deprivation may vary between types of resource, geographical location within a city, countries, and time periods.

A case study: food deserts

Access to affordable, nutritious food has been hypothesized to be an important determinant of a healthy diet, and concern has been expressed in government publications about food deserts (Acheson, 1998; Social Exclusion Unit, 1998). Contrary to our expectations, when we examined the location of different types of retail food outlets (multiple-chain supermarkets, and convenience, specialist and discount stores) in Glasgow, and studied the price and availability of a basket of everyday foodstuffs in these stores, we found that supermarkets belonging to the big multiple chains were more likely to be found in deprived neighbourhoods, all areas had reasonable access to grocery stores, there were few price differences in staple items and, when there were price differences, foods were cheaper in poorer areas (Cummins and Macintyre, 1999, 2002). Broadly similar findings were reported from Newcastle (White et al., 2004), and nationally it was noted that overall there was no evidence of lack of access to supermarkets in poorer areas since changes in planning regulations in the 1990s (Competition Commission, 2000). Similarly and more recently, a food-mapping exercise in Scotland indicated that 'there is an extensive network of food shops across all socioeconomic environments in Scotland' (Dawson et al., 2008: 2). It seems thus that, in the UK at least, a simple lack of access to food stores is not the major explanation for poorer diet and nutrition in more deprived neighbourhoods.

This suggests that we need to look for more nuanced and dynamic analyses for reasons for neighbourhood differences in diet. As White et al. (2004: 24) noted in relation to their study in Newcastle,

> In answer to the question, 'do food deserts exist?' the answer must be 'only for some'. And that 'some' is a minority of people who, for a variety of reasons, do not or cannot shop outside their immediate locality, and for whom this locality suffers from poor retail provision of foods that make up a 'healthy' diet. Our finding that the key predictors of healthy eating overall are dietary knowledge and a healthier lifestyle, must lead us to question whether those people whose diet is 'less healthy' than desirable would eat more healthily if supplied with improved retail provision. Our study does not provide evidence to support retail provision as a primary cause of consuming an 'unhealthy' diet, although poor retail provision may be an important contributing factor in some,

well defined, circumstances (e.g. when individuals are dependent on local retail provision and that provision is less than ideal).

Although a study in Leeds reported improved diets following the opening of a new supermarket in a deprived area (Wrigley et al., 2002), a study investigating food purchasing and consumption in two very deprived neighbourhoods (Shettleston and Springburn) in Glasgow before and after a major food superstore opened in Springburn (which had not previously had one), found that there was a minimal improvement in fruit and vegetable consumption between the baseline and follow-up surveys, but this did not differ between the two neighbourhoods (a finding which illustrates the importance of having a comparison group in such studies) (Cummins et al., 2005; Cummins, Findlay, Higgins et al., 2008; Cummins, Findlay, Petticrew and Sparks, 2008).

How residents themselves view local provision may be important. One UK study found that few low-income participants said that they experienced any difficulty visiting supermarkets, or perceived any problems in the choice of shops, or of fruit and vegetables, in their local area (Dibsdall et al., 2003); another study, in Hackney, London, reported that residents viewed their local provision to be poorer than a neighbouring wealthier neighbourhood (Bowyer et al., 2006). A study in Portsmouth, England, found that consumers' characteristics and circumstances can significantly reduce a broad theoretical provision of food stores to a limited set of perceived real choices (Kirkup et al., 2004). In-depth interviews with local residents as part of the Glasgow study revealed issues of boundaries and ownership: although the new superstore was located in the electoral ward of Springburn, local lay definitions of Springburn were often much narrower and sometimes situated the store outwith these boundaries. Many participants believed it to be relatively expensive compared to local stores, and some felt that the range it stocked was so large that they might be tempted to spend beyond their means. The Scottish-wide study of retail provision noted that there was a tendency for the more deprived urban areas to have a higher network density of small stores that, individually, had lower levels of availability of 'healthy eating' items and the greatest proportion of fruit and vegetables items rated as poor quality (Dawson et al., 2008).

There are also issues such as the quality of produce and in-store promotions (e.g. buy one get one free) which focus on unhealthy products (National Consumer Council, 2005). The number of such promotions seems to have increased; a study in 2008 found 17 per cent more in-store promotions than in 2006, and 83 per cent more than in 2005. Fatty and sugary foods accounted for over half of all price promotions in the leading UK retailers surveyed (Yates, 2008).

Other recent commentators have suggested that the factors affecting access to a healthy diet are multiple and extend well beyond spatial or geographical aspects and that a 'typology of food deserts' may be more useful (Shaw, 2006). Shaw (2006) proposes that the concept of 'access' may be broken down into three contributory factors: ability problems, asset problems and attitude problems. 'Ability problems' are defined as anything which physically prevents access to food which a consumer otherwise has the financial resources to purchase and the mental desire to buy, 'asset problems' are defined as the lack of financial and other means (including storage and cooking facilities) to consume food which the individual can otherwise physically access and has the desire to consume, while 'attitude problems' refer to any state of mind that prevents the consumer from accessing foods they can otherwise physically bring into their home and have the necessary assets to procure.

Conclusion

Our studies of the distribution of resources, and the research reported in the above case study on food deserts, suggests that we need to look beyond the mere location of amenities and resources in order to explain geographical inequalities in health. We can identify a number of key issues.

First, what may be important is not the objective presence of a facility, but subjective perceptions not only of its presence but its availability to the beholder. Recent work on proximity to physical activity resources has shown little agreement between objective and subjective definitions of availability (Ball et al., 2008; Macintyre et al., 2008b) and the Springburn study showed that some people did not think the new supermarket was in their locality. It may be that even if you know about a facility in your immediate neighbourhood, you need not think it is symbolically or socially suitable or accessible for yourself.

Second, even though various facilities and amenities may be equitably located across more and less deprived areas, those in poorer areas may be of worse quality. For example a study of children's play areas in Glasgow found that, although these were more likely to be located in poorer areas (Ellaway et al., 2007), safety and aesthetics were poorer in deprived areas, with more litter, broken glass, inadequate safety surfacing and rusty or broken equipment compared to play areas in more affluent areas (Hughes et al., 2008). Across Scotland, 45 per cent of people living in more deprived areas reported that a lack of safe play areas was a serious problem in their local area compared with 4 per cent of those living in the most affluent areas, and these reports may relate more to perceptions of safety and quality than actual presence or absence of facilities (Curtice et al., 2005).

Third, more general features of the social and physical environment may contribute to health inequalities. Incivilities such as litter, graffiti, vandalism and anti-social behaviour are consistently more commonly reported in poorer areas. In turn, they, together with the reputation of an area and prevailing levels of social capital and social cohesion, can be associated not only with poorer mental health but with barriers to health-enhancing behaviours such as social participation or physical activity (Sooman and Macintyre, 1995; Macintyre and Ellaway, 1999, 2000; Ellaway et al., 2001; Curtice et al., 2005).

Fourth, variations in the use and significance of the neighbourhood can be socially structured, for example by gender, age, ethnicity and social class (Kwan, 1999). The gendered experience and consequences of place for health and health behaviours have recently been noted (Molinari et al., 1998; Ellaway and Macintyre, 2001). We have found, for example, that perceptions of the provision of neighbourhood amenities seem to be more strongly associated with women's than with men's smoking status, whereas the perceived quality of the local neighbourhood appears to be a better predictor of men's smoking (Ellaway and Macintyre, 2009).

Fifth, the relevant spatial size, and the extent of differences between neighbourhoods, may vary by cultural context. For example, much of the literature on neighbourhood differences in health and health behaviours shows much more marked differences between neighbourhoods in the USA than elsewhere, probably because of much stronger patterns of racial and socio-economic segregation in the USA (Williams and Collins, 2001; Cummins and Macintyre, 2006). Given generally high population densities in European cities compared to those in North America or Australasia, neighbourhoods studied in Europe may be geographically much smaller than those elsewhere (Antrop, 2004; Kasanko et al., 2006).

To conclude, the timing of neighbourhood exposures is important too. Some aspects of the residential environment might have immediate impact upon health behaviours and outcomes (e.g. access to fruit and vegetables might influence diet) while others might have a more long-term impact (e.g. weight gain arising from a poor diet over many years). However, most studies are cross-sectional and therefore unable to shed light on the plausible timing of exposures, that is, when area influences on health are likely to be discernable in health outcomes (Macintyre et al., 2002).

Acknowledgements

Sally Macintyre and Anne Ellaway are employed by the UK Medical Research Council. This work is part of the Social & Spatial Patterning of

Health Programme (wbs 1300.00.006) at the MRC Social and Public Health Sciences Unit, Glasgow, Scotland.

References

Acheson, D. (1998) *Independent Inquiry into Inequalities in Health: Report.* London: The Stationery Office.

Antrop, M. (2004) Landscape change and the urbanization process in Europe, *Landscape and Urban Planning,* 67: 9–26.

Aveyard, P., Manaski, S. and Chambers, J. (2002) The relationship between mean birth weight and poverty using the Townsend deprivation score and the Super Profile classification system, *Public Health,* 116(6): 301–14.

Ball, K., Jeffery, R., Crawford, D. et al. (2008) Mismatch between perceived and objective measures of physical activity environments, *Preventive Medicine,* 47(3): 294–8.

Ball, K., Timperio, A.F. and Crawford, D.A. (2006) Understanding environmental influences on nutrition and physical activity behaviors: where should we look and what should we count? *International Journal of Behavioral Nutrition and Physical Activity,* 3: 1–8.

Barnard, P., Charafeddine, R., Frohlich, K., et al. (2007) Health inequalities and place: a theoretical conception of neighbourhood, *Social Science and Medicine,* 65: 1839–52.

Black, D., Morris, J., Smith, C. and Townsend, P. (1980) *Inequalities in Health: Report of a Working Party.* London: Department of Health and Social Security.

Bowyer, S., Caraher M., Duane, T. and Carr-Hill, R. (2006) *Shopping for Food: Accessing Healthy Affordable Food in Three Areas of Hackney.* London: Centre for Food Policy, City University.

Competition Commission (2000) *Supermarkets: A Report on the Supply of Groceries from Multiple Stores in the United Kingdom* (3 vols), Cm 4842. London: The Stationery Office.

Cradock, A., Kawachi, I., Colditz, G.A. et al. (2005) Playground safety and access in Boston neighbourhoods, *American Journal of Preventive Medicine,* 28: 357–63.

Cummins, S. and Macintyre, S. (1999) The location of food stores in urban areas: a case study in Glasgow, *British Food Journal,* 101: 545–53.

Cummins, S. and Macintyre, S. (2002) A systematic study of an urban foodscape: the price and availability of food in Greater Glasgow, *Urban Studies,* 39: 2115–30.

Cummins, S. and Macintyre, S. (2006) Food environments and obesity: neighbourhood or nation? *International Journal of Epidemiology,* 35: 100–4.

Cummins, S., Findlay, A., Higgins, C. et al. (2008) Reducing inequalities in health: findings from a study of the impact of a food retail development, *Environment and Planning A*, 40: 402–22.

Cummins, S., Findlay, A., Petticrew, M. and Sparks, L. (2008) Retail-led regeneration and store-switching behaviour, *Journal of Retailing and Consumer Services*, 15: 288–95.

Cummins, S., Petticrew, M., Higgins, C. et al. (2005) Large scale food retailing as an intervention for diet and health: quasi-experimental evaluation of a natural experiment, *Journal of Epidemiology and Community Health*, 59: 1035–40.

Curtice, J., Ellaway, A. and Morris, G. (2005) *Environmental Justice and Health: Results from the 2004 Scottish Social Attitudes Survey.* Edinburgh: Scottish Executive.

Dawson, J., Marshall, D., Taylor, M. et al. (2008) *Accessing Healthy Food: Sentinel Mapping Study of Healthy Food Retailing in Scotland.* Edinburgh: Food Standards Agency Scotland.

Dibsdall, L., Lambert, N., Bobbin, R. and Frewer, L. (2003) Low-income consumers' attitudes and behaviour towards access, availability and motivation to eat fruit and vegetables, *Public Health Nutrition*, 6: 159–68.

Ellaway, A., Anderson, A. and Macintyre, S. (1997) Does area of residence affect body size and shape? *International Journal of Obesity*, 21: 304–8.

Ellaway, A. and Macintyre, S. (2001) Women in their place: gender and perceptions of neighbourhoods in the West of Scotland, in I. Dyck, N. Davis Lewis and S. McLafferty (eds) *Geographies of Women's Health.* London: Routledge.

Ellaway, A. and Macintyre, S. (2009) Are perceived neighbourhood problems associated with the likelihood of smoking? *Journal of Epidemiology and Community Health*, 63: 78–80.

Ellaway, A., Kirk, A., Macintyre, S. and Mutrie, N. (2007) Nowhere to play? The relationship between the location of outdoor play areas and deprivation in Glasgow, *Health and Place*, 13: 557–61.

Ellaway, A., Macintyre, S. and Kearns, A. (2001) Perceptions of place and health in socially contrasting neighbourhoods, *Urban Studies*, 38: 2299–316.

Ellen, I.G., Mijanovich, T. and Dillman, K.-N. (2001) Neighborhood effects on health: exploring the links and assessing the evidence, *Journal of Urban Affairs*, 23: 391–408.

Flinn, M.W. (1965) *Report on the Sanitary Conditions of the Labouring Population of Great Britain by Edwin Chadwick.* Edinburgh: Edinburgh University Press.

Galster, G. (2001) On the nature of neighbourhood, *Urban Studies*, 38: 2111–24.

Giles-Corti, B. and Donovan, R.J. (2002) Socioeconomic status differences in recreational physical activity levels and real and perceived access to a supportive physical environment, *Preventive Medicine*, 35: 601–11.

Hofrichter, R. (1993) *Toxic Struggles*. Philadelphia, PA: New Society.

Hughes, C., Macintyre, S. and Mutrie, N. (2008) *Socio-economic Variations in the Quality of Play Provision in Glasgow, UK*. Symposium Presentation, International Society of Behavioural Nutrition and Physical Activity Annual Meeting, Banff, Alberta, Canada.

Kasanko, M., Barredo, J.I., Lavalle, C. et al. (2006) Are European cities becoming dispersed? A comparative analysis of 15 European urban areas, *Landscape and Urban Planning*, 77: 111–30.

Kearns, A. and Parkinson, M. (2001) The significance of neighbourhood, *Urban Studies*, 38: 2103–10.

Kirkup, M., De Kervenoael, R., Hillsworth, A. et al. (2004) Inequalities in retail choice: exploring consumer experiences in suburban neighbourhoods, *International Journal of Retail and Distribution Management*, 32: 511–22.

Kwan, M.-P. (1999) Gender and individual access to urban opportunities: a study using space-time measures, *Professional Geographer*, 51: 210–27.

Macintyre, S. (2007) *Inequalities in Health in Scotland: What Are They and What Can We Do About Them?* Occasional Paper 17. Glasgow: MRC Social and Public Health Sciences Unit.

Macintyre, S. and Ellaway, A. (1998) Social and local variations in the use of urban neighbourhoods: a case study in Glasgow, *Health and Place*, 4: 91–4.

Macintyre, S. and Ellaway, A. (1999) Local opportunity structures, social capital and social inequalities in health: what can central and local government do? *Health Promotion Journal of Australia*, 9: 165–70.

Macintyre, S. and Ellaway, A. (2000) Neighbourhood cohesion and health in socially contrasting neighbourhoods: implications for the social exclusion and public health agendas, *Health Bulletin*, 58: 450–6.

Macintyre, S. and Ellaway, A. (2003) Neighbourhoods and health: overview, in I. Kawachi and L. Berkman (eds) *Neighbourhoods and Health*. Oxford: Oxford University Press.

Macintyre, S., Ellaway, A. and Cummins, S. (2002) Place effects on health: how can we conceptualise and measure them? *Social Science and Medicine*, 55: 125–39.

Macintyre, S., MacDonald, L. and Ellaway, A. (2008a) Do poorer people have poorer access to local resources and facilities? The distribution of local resources by area deprivation in Glasgow, Scotland, *Social Science and Medicine*, 67: 900–14.

Macintyre, S., MacDonald, L. and Ellaway, A. (2008b) Lack of agreement between measured and self-reported distance from public green parks in Glasgow, Scotland, *International Journal of Behavioral Nutrition and Physical Activity*, 5: 1–8.

Macintyre, S., Maciver, S. and Sooman, A. (1993) Area, class and health: should we be focusing on places or people? *Journal of Social Policy*, 22: 213–34.

Molinari, C., Ahern, M. and Hendryx, M. (1998) The relationship of community quality to the health of women and men, *Social Science and Medicine*, 47: 1113–20.

National Consumer Council (2005) *Healthy Competition: How Supermarkets Can Affect Your Chances of a Healthy Diet*. London: National Consumer Council.

O'Campo, P., Xue, X., Wang, M.C. and Caughy, M. (1997) Neighborhood risk factors for low birthweight in Baltimore: a multilevel analysis, *American Journal of Public Health*, 87(7):1113–18.

Office for National Statistics (ONS) (2008) *Neighbourhood Statistics*. Available at: www.neighbourhood.statistics.gov.uk.

Pearce, J., Witten, K., Hiscock, R. and Blakely, T. (2007) Are socially disadvantaged neighbourhoods deprived of health-related community resources? *International Journal of Epidemiology*, 36(2): 348–55.

Pickett, K.E. and Pearl, M. (2001) Multilevel analyses of neighbourhood socio-economic context and health outcomes: a critical review, *Journal of Epidemiology and Community Health*, 55: 111–22.

Powell, L.M., Slater, S., Chaloupka, F.J. and Harper, D. (2006) Availability of physical activity-related facilities and neighborhood demographic and socioeconomic characteristics: a national study, *American Journal of Public Health*, 96: 1676–80.

Riva, M., Gauvin, L. and Barnett, T. (2007) Towards the next generation of research into small area effects on health: a synthesis of multilevel investigations published since July 1998, *Journal of Epidemiology and Community Health*, 61: 853–61.

Ross, N.A., Tremblay, S., Khan, S. et al. (2007) Body Mass Index in urban Canada: neighborhood and metropolitan area effects, *American Journal of Public Health*, 97: 500–8.

Scottish Executive (2004) *Scottish Index of Mutliple Deprivation 2004*. Available at: www.scotland.gov.uk/Publications/2005/01/20458/49127.

Sellstrom, E. and Bremberg, S. (2006) The significance of neighbourhood context to child and adolescent health and well-being: A systematic review of multilevel studies, *Scandinavian Journal of Public Health*, 34: 544–54.

Sellstrom, E., Arnoldsson, G., Bremberg, S. and Hjern, A. (2007) Are there differences in birth weight between neighbourhoods in a Nordic welfare state? *BMC Public Health*, 7: 267.

Shaw, H.J. (2006) Food deserts: Towards the development of a classification. *Geografiska Annaler Series B-Human Geography*, 88B: 231–47.

Social Exclusion Unit (1998) *Bringing Britain Together: A National Strategy for Neighbourhood Renewal*. London: Social Exclusion Unit.

Sooman, A. and Macintyre, S. (1995) Health and perceptions of the local environment in socially contrasting neighbourhoods in Glasgow, *Health and Place*, 1: 15–26.

Spencer, N., Bambang, S., Loga, S. and Gill, L. (1999) Socioeconomic status and birth weight: comparison of an area-based measure with the Registrar Generals's social class, *Journal of Epidemiology and Community Health*, 53: 495–8.

Tudor Hart, J. (1971) The inverse care law. *Lancet*, 1: 405–12.

Van Lenthe, F.J., Brug, J. and Mackenbach, J.P. (2005) Neighbourhood inequalities in physical inactivity: the role of neighbourhood attractiveness, proximity to local facilities and safety in the Netherlands, *Social Science and Medicine*, 60: 763–75.

White, M., Williams, E., Raybould, S. et al. (2004) *Do Food Deserts Exist? A Multi-level Geographical Analysis of the Relationship between Retail Food Access, Socio-economic Position and Dietary Intake*. Final report to Food Standards Agency. London: Food Standards Agency.

Williams, D.R. and Collins, C. (2001) Racial residential segregation: a fundamental cause of racial disparities in health, *Public Health Reports*, 116: 404–16.

Winkler, E., Turrell, G. and Patterson, C. (2006) Does living in a disadvantaged area entail limited opportunities to purchase fresh fruit and vegetables in terms of price, availability, and variety? Findings from the Brisbane Food Study, *Health and Place*, 12: 741–8.

Wrigley, N., Warm, D., Margetts, B. and Whelan, A. (2002) Assessing the impact of improved retail access on diet in a 'food desert': a preliminary report, *Urban Studies*, 39: 2061–82.

Yates, L. (2008) *Cut-price, What Cost? How Supermarkets Can Affect Your Chances of a Healthy Diet*. London: National Consumer Council.

Zenk, S., Schulz, A., Israel, B. et al. (2005) Neighborhood racial composition, neighborhood poverty, and the spatial accessibility of supermarkets in metropolitan Detroit, *American Journal of Public Health*, 95: 660–7.

Part 2

Health inequalities: understanding intersections

Part 2 is framed by an appreciation that socio-economic inequality is only one of a spectrum of inequalities influencing people's lives and people's health. Such an appreciation is particularly important in societies like the UK which are distinguished by persisting inequalities between men and women and between ethnic and religious groups.

The chapters focus on ethnicity, religion, disability, gender and age to illustrate the multiple dimensions of people's identity and how these multiple identities shape, and are shaped by, their socio-economic position. Drawing on both quantitative and qualitative research, the authors note that identities are not fixed and 'set in concrete'; they are constantly being negotiated as we grow up, make our way through key transitions on the pathway to adulthood and go about our adult lives. Linking the chapters, too, is an emphasis on how wider society influences the expression of identity and the realization of ambitions, with disadvantaged groups seeking to assert a positive sense of self in the face of prejudice and discrimination.

Two chapters focus on ethnicity and religion, and how these intersect with each other and with other dimensions of identity and inequality. James Nazroo and Saffron Karlsen turn to quantitative studies to discuss the intersections between ethnicity, religion and socio-economic position. Karl Atkin draws on qualitative research to illuminate how ethnicity and religion influence, and are expressed through, the experiences of young people with impairments and adults at risk of haemoglobin disorders.

Two chapters focus on the intersections between gender and socio-economic inequality. In Kate Hunt and David Batty's chapter, quantitative studies are the major source of evidence on the socio-economic patterning of health and health behaviour among men and women. Naomi Rudoe and Rachel Thomson draw primarily on qualitative studies of young people to deepen understanding of how socio-economic advantage and disadvantage influence the experience of gender and, thereby, the meanings attached to early parenthood.

2.1 Religion, ethnicity and health inequalities

Saffron Karlsen and James Nazroo

Introduction

Differences in health across ethnic/race groups have been repeatedly documented. Ethnic differences are found in the UK (Erens et al., 2001), the USA (Williams, 2001), Latin America (Pan American Health Organization, 2001), South Africa (Sidiropoulos et al., 1997), Australia (McLennan and Madden 1999), New Zealand (Harris et al., 2006) and elsewhere. There is now convincing evidence that social and economic inequalities underpin much of the observed ethnic/racial inequality in health (Nazroo and Williams, 2005). However, other dimensions of social identity that might be racialized, such as religious affiliation, have not been much investigated.

In the first edition of *Understanding Health Inequalities* (Karlsen and Nazroo, 2000), we argued that theorizing ethnicity as a social identity was an important starting point for an investigation of inequalities in health. In part, the importance of identity comes from the cultural location and the cultural resources that it offers, which map onto health-related behaviours and which locate individuals within communities that may provide material resources and social resources (like social networks, support, opportunities for participation etc.). But such social identities have the potential to also operate as markers of boundaries between groups, boundaries that may be imposed and that may have both symbolic and material consequences for those who are, and are not, members of the group. These processes have clear implications for health, suggesting that it would be fruitful to examine both processes of identification with minority identities, and the consequences of being identified as a member of a minority group. While work on this has progressed in relation to ethnicity and race, the role of religious identities has generally been neglected. Yet, in contemporary societies it seems likely that religious identities, particularly minority religious identities, can provide social locations that offer social resources, but they may also be identities that are racialized with consequent negative social and economic consequences.

In this chapter, we set out to explore the intersection of religious and ethnic identities in the UK, and how this relates to both health and the underlying social and economic inequalities that might drive any health inequality. The variability of ethnic and religious categories in the UK and the ways in which they intersect, together with a large literature on ethnic inequalities in health, gives great potential for such research. The neglect of religious identities in the health inequalities field has, at least in part, been a consequence of the lack of suitable data. Until the introduction of a question on religion at the 2001 Census, there had been no population-level data to explore the circumstances of different religious groups. A small number of UK surveys also include information on religious identities. In analyses of the *Fourth National Survey of Ethnic Minorities* (FNS), there was some investigation of differences in health by religious groups among the Indian ethnic category, which suggested that Muslim Indians had poorer health than Sikh and Hindu Indians (Nazroo, 2001). But the more recent data from the 1999 and 2004 *Health Survey for England*, both of which contained a boosted ethnic minority sample, have not been used in this way. Consequently, this chapter presents a novel, but initial, examination of the relationships between health and ethnic and religious identity.

Data sources and content

Data from the UK Census 2001 are used to provide background information on the size of different religious and ethnic groups in the UK. We use the *Health Survey for England* (HSE) to examine differences in health across ethnic/religious groups, combining data from the 1999 (Erens et al., 2001) and 2004 (Sproston and Mindell, 2006) sweeps to maximize sample sizes. We also make use of data from *EMPIRIC*, a follow-up survey of the HSE 1999 that included the collection of data on mental health and on experiences and perceptions of racism and discrimination.

The Health Survey for England (HSE)

The HSE is a series of nationally representative surveys about the health of people in England that has been conducted annually since 1991. In 1999 and 2004, the focus of the HSE was on the health of ethnic minority people, with boosted samples of Irish, Black Caribbean, Indian, Pakistani, Bangladeshi and Chinese respondents. The 2004 HSE additionally had a boosted sample of Black African respondents. Respondents were allocated into ethnic categories on the basis of their response to a question asking about family origins. They were also asked to identify their religion, or church.

To cover different regions and socio-economic profiles, respondents were recruited from addresses selected from within a sample of postcode sectors that were stratified using Census data (1991 Census for the 1999 survey and 2001 Census for the 2004 survey). For the ethnic minority samples, postcode sectors were also stratified and selected on the basis of their ethnic composition. Areas with low concentrations of ethnic minority people were identified and included, but in these areas screening for respondents used the focused enumeration technique, which has been shown to produce unbiased samples (Smith and Prior, 1997). The Chinese population is more geographically dispersed than other groups, so was sampled by screening addresses where information from the electoral register indicated that one or more of the residents had a Chinese origin name (the detail of this procedure varied between the 1999 and 2004 surveys). Sample sizes for the ethnic minority groups included in the surveys are: Caribbean 2362, Black African 859, Indian 2467, Bangladeshi 1985, Pakistani 2204, Chinese 1385 and Irish 2398. Full details of the sample design can be found in the survey reports (Erens et al., 2001; Sproston and Mindell, 2006).

Survey materials were translated into five languages (Hindi, Gujarati, Punjabi, Urdu and Bengali) by an experienced independent professional translation service. The interview was carried out in the language(s) of the respondent's choice by a bilingual interviewer.

EMPIRIC

EMPIRIC involved a follow-up survey of respondents to the HSE 1999. It included those who were Caribbean, Indian, Pakistani, Bangladeshi, Irish or white British, aged 16–74 years, and had agreed to be recontacted (92% of those eligible) (for full details, see Sproston and Nazroo, 2002). The overall response rate for the *EMPIRIC* study was 68.2 per cent, with some variation across the ethnic groups (ranging from 62% of Indian people to 72% of Irish people). Sample sizes for the *EMPIRIC* survey are: Caribbean 695, Indian 641, Bangladeshi 650, Pakistani 724, Irish 733 and white British 838. Weights were developed to adjust for non-response, taking advantage of our ability to model non-response using data collected at the HSE 1999 interview. Full details of the sample design can be found in Sproston and Nazroo (2002).

Measures

Ethnicity was categorized using responses to a question on family origins, which has a strong correlation with Census ethnic identity categories (Nazroo, 2001). The following categories are used in the analyses of

HSE data: white British, Caribbean, Indian, Pakistani, Bangladeshi, Black African, Chinese and Irish. For the analyses of *EMPIRIC* data, the categories are restricted to: Caribbean, Indian, Pakistani, Bangladeshi, Irish and white British.

Religion was categorized using responses to a question that asked, 'What is your religion or church?'. Categories used are: Christian, Muslim, Hindu, Sikh, Buddhist and none. The analyses that we present examine the intersection of ethnic and religious categories, so we compare different religious groups, different ethnic groups within religious categories, and different religions within ethnic categories.

To cover demographic and socio-economic circumstances, we used data on age, gender and a range of socio-economic measures (see Hilary Graham's introductory chapter on the measurement of socio-economic position). The measures were employment status, occupational class (household social class using the Registrar General's occupational classification), housing tenure, highest formal educational qualification and household income (collected in categories using a showcard), which was equivalized using the standard scoring system to take account of the number of people in the household and categorized into population-specific quintiles.

The *EMPIRIC* study contained three measures of exposure to racist victimization over the previous year, covering verbal abuse, a physical attack, or damage to their property. These were combined to represent those who had been racially victimized and those who had not. Respondents were also asked whether they had ever been refused a job, or been treated unfairly with regard to a promotion or move to a better position at work, for reasons which they believed were related to their race, colour or their religious or ethnic background. Again, the indicators were combined. There is evidence that racism can influence an individual's well-being even in the absence of personal experiences of racist victimization (Karlsen and Nazroo, 2004). To explore this, we included responses to a question asking what proportion of British employers the respondent believed would discriminate when recruiting. This indicator was dichotomized to distinguish between those who perceived none or a few and those who perceived half or more British employers to discriminate.

Health was assessed using a combination of global self-reports, symptom reports, reports of diagnosed conditions, and direct measures. Self-reports included self-assessed general health (comparing 'very good' or 'good', with 'fair', 'poor' or 'very poor'), and the presence of an activity-limiting long-standing illness. Symptom reports were used to measure common mental disorders, using the Revised Clinical Interview Schedule (CIS-R; Lewis et al., 1992). This instrument collects data on the presence and severity of 14 non-psychotic psychiatric symptoms during the week prior to interview, including those of anxiety and depression, which can then be used to indicate the presence or absence of a common mental disorder (Lewis et al., 1992). Reported diagnoses covered hypertension and diabetes. The direct measure of health included here is waist–hip ratio, which is a measure of central obesity. It is considered a more useful measure than body mass index when comparing ethnic groups, because it more clearly distinguishes body fat from body shape. Waist and hip measures were taken during a nurse visit to the respondent and the ratio is calculated as waist circumference divided by hip circumference (mm). Although there is no complete consensus about the threshold of waist–hip ratio that indicates increased risk (Molarius and Seidell, 1998), we used commonly recognized indicators for women (> 0.85) and men (> 0.95).

Sample weights

Both the 1999 and 2004 HSE samples had a boosted ethnic minority component, which meant that the sample had to be weighted to correct for the unequal probabilities of selection for different classes of respondents (see Erens et al., 2001; Sproston and Mindell, 2006, for details). As the *EMPIRIC* sample was drawn from the HSE 1999, additional weights were applied to adjust for non-response to the *EMPIRIC* survey (see Sproston and Nazroo, 2002, for details). In addition, for both studies, the stratified and clustered nature of the sample design meant that standard errors were also corrected for auto-correlation within the stratified multi-stage design.

Ethnic and religious make-up of the UK population

At the 2001 Census, 7.9 per cent of the UK population (just over 4.6 million people) identified themselves as members of a non-white ethnic minority group, with an additional 1.2 per cent identifying as white Irish and 2.5 per cent as 'other white' in Great Britain (the collection of white minority categories was not included in the Census of Northern Ireland). Of the non-white minority groups, 23 per cent described themselves as Indian, 16 per cent as Pakistani, 6 per cent as Bangladeshi, 12 per cent as Black Caribbean, 10 per cent as Black African, 5 per cent as Chinese, 15 per cent as mixed, and the rest as a member of one of the 'other' categories.

A similarly small proportion of the population described themselves as having a religion other than Christian. Seventy-two per cent of the population described themselves as Christian, 15 per cent said they had no religion, 8 per cent did not answer this question (it was voluntary), and 5.4 per cent chose a non-Christian religion. Of the non-Christian religious categories, Muslim was the most commonly chosen, with 52 per cent of this population, 18 per cent described themselves as Hindu, 11 per cent

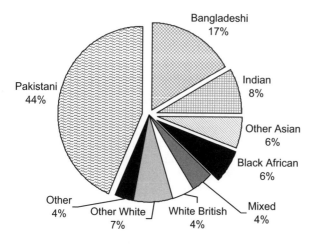

Figure 2.1.1 The ethnic make-up of the UK Muslim population, 2001 Census.

as Sikh, 9 per cent as Jewish and 5 per cent as Buddhist, with 5 per cent choosing another religion.

Some of these religious categories map reasonably clearly onto ethnic categories, but an examination of the ethnic make-up of the Muslim category, shown in Figure 2.1.1, indicates the obvious potential for diversity within religious categories. Similarly, while some ethnic categories map reasonably clearly onto religious categories, an examination of the religious make-up of the Indian population (including a significant proportion of each of Hindu, Muslim, Sikh and Christian) indicates the potential for diversity within ethnic categories.

The intersection between ethnicity and religion in the data used here (from the HSE), is shown in Table 2.1.1. While this reflects the position of the ethnic groups included in the HSE, that study did not include all ethnic groups.

Religious and ethnic differences in health

We examined relative levels of health for different religious and ethnic groups using five markers of health, which covered self-reported health status, diagnosed conditions and raised waist–hip ratio (a direct measure of health). Findings are shown in Table 2.1.2. The table contrasts the health of six religious groups (Christian minority, no religion, Muslim, Sikh, Hindu and Buddhist) with a white Christian group, and also considers ethnic categories within three of these categories of religion (Christian

Table 2.1.1 Ethnic breakdown of religious groups

	Column per cents					
	No religion	*Christian*	*Buddhist*	*Muslim*	*Hindu*	*Sikh*
White British	94	94	65	9	2	0
Irish	2	4	4	0	0	0
Black Caribbean	1	1	1	1	0	0
Black African	0	1	0	9	0	0
Chinese	1	0	28	0	0	0
Indian	0	0	3	12	97	100
Pakistani	0	0	0	50	0	0
Bangladeshi	0	0	0	20	0	0
Base	*3969*	*15848*	*290*	*4651*	*1197*	*657*

minority, no religion and Muslim). The first row of the table shows the prevalence of these conditions for white Christian people, while the rest of the table shows the age and gender standardized odds ratios for specific groups to have each of the conditions compared with white Christians.

The most striking finding in the table is that the health of the white Christian group is as good as, or better than, all of the other religious/ethnic categories. For the six health conditions and 17 religious/ethnic minority categories examined, the table contains 85 comparisons with the white Christian group. Of these, there are only five instances where the health of the minority group is significantly better than that of white Christians: Black African and Chinese Christians, and Chinese people with no religion, had a significantly lower rate of limiting long-standing illness; and Chinese people with no religion and Buddhists had a lower rate of hypertension. In contrast, in 38 of the 85 comparisons, the health of the religious minority group is worse than that of white Christians. This is most obviously the case for two religious categories – Muslim and Sikh – and one ethnic category – Caribbean. Each of the Muslim groups (Pakistani, Bangladeshi and Indian) had a significantly higher risk of each of the conditions apart from hypertension, and the level of the increased risk seems similar across each of the Muslim groups. The Sikh group had an increased risk for each of these conditions (including hypertension) compared with the white Christian group, although for several conditions this increased risk was not as great as that for the Muslim groups (hypertension was the exception to this). Increased risks were also present for most conditions for the Caribbean Christian and Caribbean no religion groups (for limiting longstanding illness the difference for

Table 2.1.2 Religious and ethnic differences in health

	Fair/poor self-assessed health	Limiting long-standing illness	Diagnosed diabetes	Diagnosed hypertension	Raised waist–hip ratio
	Age and gender standardized odds-ratio (95% C.I.) compared with white Christian				
White Christian*	1.00 (26%)	1.00 (27%)	1.00 (4%)	1.00 (19%)	1.00 (30%)
Christian minority					
All	1.22 (1.05,1.42)	1.01 (0.88,1.17)	1.28 (0.71,2.31)	1.09 (0.81,1.47)	1.27 (1.02,1.58)
Irish	1.09 (0.91,1.31)	1.06 (0.90,1.25)	0.78 (0.41,1.51)	1.04 (0.76,1.42)	1.35 (1.03,1.77)
Black Caribbean	2.04 (1.75,2.38)	1.18 (0.99,1.39)	3.48 (1.93,6.27)	1.79 (1.32,2.43)	1.72 (1.31,2.26)
Black African	0.84 (0.47,1.50)	0.48 (0.28,0.83)	2.02 (0.88,4.66)	1.34 (0.88,2.02)	1.83 (1.12,2.97)
Chinese	0.65 (0.39,1.08)	0.36 (0.21,0.61)	1.55 (0.68,3.50)	0.87 (0.55,1.38)	1.03 (0.67,1.59)
Indian	0.92 (0.57,1.51)	0.73 (0.43,1.24)	2.28 (0.86,6.03)	1.11 (0.61,2.02)	2.29 (1.17,4.48)
No religion					
All	1.01 (0.90,1.16)	0.96 (0.84,1.09)	1.68 (0.84,3.37)	0.97 (0.65,1.43)	0.80 (0.52,1.24)
White British	1.00 (0.88,1.15)	0.97 (0.86,1.11)	1.29 (0.21,7.88)	0.38 (0.14,1.05)	0.51 (0.24,1.08)
Chinese	0.88 (0.54,1.45)	0.25 (0.16,0.38)	1.69 (0.83,3.44)	0.47 (0.31,0.70)	1.05 (0.70,1.59)
Caribbean	2.04 (1.50,2.77)	1.58 (1.15,2.17)	4.48 (1.97,10.16)	1.47 (0.93,2.31)	1.39 (0.76,2.55)
Muslim					
All	2.48 (2.05,2.99)	1.35 (1.09,1.66)	5.34 (2.96,9.64)	1.04 (0.76,1.42)	2.92 (2.22,3.83)
Pakistani	2.26 (1.94,2.64)	1.42 (1.21,1.67)	5.00 (2.73,9.16)	1.23 (0.89,1.68)	3.12 (2.31,4.22)
Bangladeshi	2.94 (2.52,3.43)	1.49 (1.27,1.76)	5.48 (2.99,10.05)	0.86 (0.60,1.22)	4.09 (2.93,5.71)
Indian	2.68 (1.91,3.76)	1.70 (1.18,2.45)	6.33 (2.86,14.00)	0.84 (0.52,1.36)	2.71 (1.78,4.12)
Sikh	2.17 (1.67,2.80)	1.50 (1.10,2.04)	3.18 (1.65,6.13)	1.53 (1.06,2.19)	2.69 (1.90,3.80)
Hindu	1.59 (1.30,1.94)	0.79 (0.59,1.06)	2.96 (1.56,5.61)	0.98 (0.69,1.40)	1.37 (1.03,1.82)
Buddhist	2.41 (1.36,4.26)	1.72 (0.89,3.33)	1.26 (0.31,5.09)	0.29 (0.12,0.75)	1.54 (0.80,2.97)

*White British and other white groups, excluding Irish people, prevalence is shown in brackets.

Caribbean Christians was only statistically significant at the $p < 0.1$ level). Again, however, the odds were on average not quite as high as those for the Muslim groups.

In contrast with Indian Muslims and Sikhs, the health of Indian Christians and of Hindus compared relatively favourably with that of white Christians. Indian Christians had a higher risk of a raised waist–hip ratio, and Hindus had a higher risk of fair or poor self-assessed health, raised waist–hip ratio and of diabetes. In each case, however, the risks were not as high as those for Muslims or Sikhs. In only one case did the Chinese Christian, Chinese no-religion, or Buddhist group have a higher risk of poorer health than white Christians – for Buddhists and fair or poor self-assessed health – and, as described earlier, in four cases their health was significantly better. The health of Black African Christians was significantly worse than that of white Christians in only one case (raised waist–hip ratio) and significantly better in one case (limiting long-standing illness). Differences for the other two groups, Irish Christians and white with no religion, compared with the white Christian group were small and only significant in one case (the higher risk of raised waist-hip ratio for Irish Christians).

Although this description of differences in health across religious and ethnic groups adds to our understanding of how health varies across the population, it does not give an indication of why such differences might emerge. Elsewhere we have provided evidence to suggest that the social and economic inequalities associated with an ethnic minority identity, including experiences of racism and discrimination, drive ethnic inequalities in health (Nazroo, 2001, 2003; Karlsen and Nazroo, 2002, 2004; Nazroo and Williams, 2005). The next section considers the patterning of such inequalities across the religious and ethnic groups that we are studying here.

Social position and experiences and perceptions of racism and discrimination

Five markers of socio-economic position are considered here: having no qualifications, living in a household headed by a manual worker, being registered unemployed, being unemployed or long-term sick, and living in a household in the bottom income quintile. Table 2.1.3 shows the distribution of these markers by religious and ethnic group. The white Christian, all minority Christian and Irish Christian groups have very similar socio-economic profiles. The Indian Christian group and, particularly, the Chinese Christian groups have a better profile than the other Christian groups. The Chinese Christian group have a better profile than all others

Table 2.1.3 Religious and ethnic differences in socio-economic position

	No qualifi-cations	Manual occupation	Registered unemployed	Unemployed or long-term sick	Bottom income quintile
	Cell percentages				
White Christian*	33	48	2	6	18
Christian minority					
All	29	48	3	8	23
Irish	33	48	2	8	19
Black Caribbean	34	56	5	11	35
Black African	14	40	4	8	30
Chinese	18	23	1	2	8
Indian	15	30	3	5	18
No religion					
All	18	40	3	6	14
White British	18	39	3	6	14
Chinese	24	51	7	8	25
Caribbean	24	47	8	15	37
Muslim					
All	42	56	7	12	51
Pakistani	44	61	6	12	52
Bangladeshi	52	74	9	13	73
Indian	37	53	4	9	51
Sikh	38	64	2	7	38
Hindu	25	32	3	7	22
Buddhist	26	46	2	6	28

*White British and other white groups, excluding Irish people.

on each of the markers. The Indian Christian group had fewer people with no qualifications or in a manual occupation (as do white British people with no religion). The Hindu group also has a better profile, although not to the same extent as the Indian Christian group and with a slightly worse income profile. The Buddhist and Black African Christian groups have a good profile in some respects (comparatively low proportions with no qualifications and in manual occupations), but a worse profile in relation to income. Black Caribbean Christians and Sikhs have a higher proportion in manual occupations and almost two-fifths of them are in the bottom income quintile. However, as for health, the Muslim groups have the worst profile. There are some differences between the Muslim groups, with Indian Muslims in a better position than Pakistani Muslims on all markers except income, where half of both groups are in the bottom

Table **2.1.4** Religious and ethnic differences in experiences of racism and perceptions of discrimination

	Racial victimization in the past year	Discrimination at work (ever)	Believe half or more British employers discriminate
Christian or no religion			
Irish	8	9	14
Black Caribbean	15	39	38
Indian	6	21	4
Muslim	12	21	19
Sikh	15	21	23
Hindu	11	23	23

quintile. Across all markers, the Bangladeshi Muslim group have by far the worst profile. For example, almost three-quarters of the Bangladeshi Muslim group are in the bottom income quintile.

Experiences of racism, discrimination at work, and perceptions of the extent of discrimination among employers in Britain are shown in Table 2.1.4 for the religious/ethnic groups included in the *EMPIRIC* study. The smaller sample sizes in that study mean that the Muslim group could not be separated into its sub-components (Bangladeshi, Indian and Pakistani), and the Christian and no religion groups are combined. For the measures reflecting experiences of victimisation and of discrimination, Table 2.1.4 shows that those in the Black Caribbean group reported the highest rates, with the Muslim, Sikh and Hindu groups having the next highest rates. The Indian Christian/no religion group had a lower rate of experienced victimization, while the Irish Christian/no religion group had a lower rate of both victimization and discrimination at work. Perceptions of the extent of discrimination by British employers followed a similar pattern to those of experiences of discrimination and victimization, although the Indian Christian/no religion group had a particularly low rate.

Religion, socio-economic position and health

Table 2.1.5 gives an indication of the potential impact of socio-economic disadvantage on health. It shows the odds ratios (and 95% confidence intervals) associated with decreasing income quintiles for the five health outcomes shown in Table 2.1.2 and for each religious/ethnic group. The

Table 2.1.5 Income gradient in health outcomes

	Fair/poor self-assessed health	Limiting long-standing illness	Diagnosed diabetes	Diagnosed hypertension	Raised waist–hip ratio
	Age and gender standardized odds-ratio (95% C.I.) for each decline in income quintile				
White Christian*	1.47 (1.40,1.54)	1.28 (1.23,1.34)	1.01 (0.60,1.69)	1.19(0.98,1.46)	1.13 (0.94,1.37)
Christian minority					
All	1.61 (1.45,1.78)	1.31 (1.18,1.45)	1.23 (1.03,1.48)	1.11 (1.00,1.23)	1.17 (1.06,1.29)
Irish	1.74 (1.53,1.99)	1.30 (1.14,1.47)	1.17 (0.85,1.59)	1.13 (0.99,1.29)	1.17 (1.03,1.32)
Black Caribbean	1.39 (1.22,1.57)	1.40 (1.21,1.62)	1.10 (0.87,1.39)	0.94 (0.82,1.07)	1.20 (1.01,1.43)
Black African	1.32(0.88,1.97)	1.76 (1.21,2.57)	1.14 (0.73,1.79)	1.07 (0.87,1.33)	0.93 (0.69,1.26)
Chinese	1.66 (1.23,2.24)	1.41 (1.00,1.980)	1.17 (0.79,1.73)	0.97 (0.76,1.25)	0.94 (0.69,1.28)
Indian	1.45 (0.85,2.47)	1.48 (0.82,2.66)	1.57 (0.46,5.42)	1.53 (0.89,2.64)	1.97 (0.99,3.93)
No religion					
All	1.46 (1.33,1.60)	1.26 (1.16,1.37)	1.71 (1.28,2.27)	1.26 (1.02,1.56)	1.28 (1.00,1.64)
White British	1.45 (1.32,1.61)	1.24 (1.14,1.36)	—	0.74 (0.43,1.28)	1.33 (0.77,2.25)
Chinese	1.49 (1.18,1.88)	1.74 (1.25,2.43)	1.01 (0.67,1.53)	1.37 (1.00,1.86)	1.14 (0.91,1.44)
Caribbean	1.56 (1.21,2.01)	1.33 (1.04,1.72)	1.88 (0.92,3.81)	1.05 (0.78,1.42)	1.38 (0.90,2.12)
Muslim					
All	1.35 (1.10,1.64)	1.52 (1.25,1.85)	1.10 (0.92,1.32)	1.08 (0.92,1.26)	1.15 (1.01,1.30)
Pakistani	1.61 (1.37,1.89)	1.31 (1.12,1.53)	1.19 (0.91,1.56)	1.07 (0.92,1.25)	1.03 (0.89,1.20)
Bangladeshi	1.21 (0.99,1.48)	1.14 (0.91,1.43)	1.17 (0.61,2.25)	1.29 (0.69,2.43)	1.06 (0.78,1.43)
Indian	1.56 (1.05,2.31)	1.90 (1.21,2.98)	1.36 (0.92,1.99)	1.22 (0.68,2.20)	1.39 (0.92,2.10)
Sikh	1.25 (0.97,1.60)	1.44 (1.08,1.92)	1.22 (0.74,1.99)	1.02 (0.81,1.29)	1.51 (1.18,1.91)
Hindu	1.15 (0.98,1.35)	1.33 (1.08,1.63)	1.32 (1.04,1.69)	1.10 (0.93,1.30)	1.12 (0.96,1.32)
Buddhist	1.52 (1.00,2.32)	0.88 (0.50,1.56)	0.69 (0.30,1.59)	0.90 (0.56,1.45)	1.81 (1.16,2.82)

*White British and other white groups, excluding Irish people, prevalence is shown in brackets.

odds ratios shown are for those in a particular income quintile relative to the odds for those belonging to the next richer quintile, so an odds ratio above 1 indicates decreasing health with decreasing income. The estimate is obtained by treating the income quintile measure as a continuous variable in a logistic regression equation, so the technique assumes that the relative odds are the same whether one is comparing the poorest and next poorest quintiles, or the second richest and richest quintiles. This assumption does not hold entirely, of course, but the figure obtained with this technique does provide an acceptable summary of the size and significance of the income gradient.

The clear impression from Table 2.1.5 is of marked and statistically significant inequalities in health for all outcomes and in each group. Of the 90 odds ratios representing income gradients in health in the table, almost half (43) are greater than 1 to a statistically significant degree (indicating that poorer health is significantly associated with lower incomes), and only 8 are less than 1 (and none of these are significantly less than 1). Those groups with larger sample sizes are more likely to have significant results: all five odds ratios are significant for the all Christian minority and all no religion groups; three are significant for the all Muslim and Sikh groups; and two odds ratios are significant for the white Christian, Hindu and Buddhist groups. Comparing the health outcomes, almost all odds are significant for self-assessed health and limiting long-standing illness, while only a few are significant for diabetes and hypertension, with raised waist–hip ratio somewhere between. Larger sample sizes would be needed to adequately test whether differences across religious/ethnic groups and health outcomes were meaningful.

Although Table 2.1.5 shows the presence of socio-economic inequalities for a range of health outcomes within each of these religious/ethnic groups, we cannot conclude from this that they contribute to the inequalities we have described across religious/ethnic groups. The examination of the contribution of socio-economic inequalities to ethnic inequalities in health involves including socio-economic measures in a regression model predicting health outcomes, in order to control for any socio-economic differences across the groups being compared. This approach is beset with problems, however, because it assumes that the socio-economic measures used are comprehensive and equivalent across the groups being compared. As Kaufman et al. (1998) point out, the process of standardization is effectively an attempt to deal with the non-random nature of samples used in cross-sectional population studies: controlling for all relevant 'extraneous' explanatory factors introduces the *appearance* of randomization. But attempting to introduce randomization into cross-sectional studies by adding 'controls' has a number of problems, summarised by Kaufman et al. (1998: 147) in the following way:

> When considering socio-economic exposures and making com-
> parisons between racial/ethnic groups . . . the material, behavioral,
> and psychological circumstances of diverse socio-economic and
> racial/ethnic groups are distinct on so many dimensions that no
> realistic adjustment can plausibly simulate randomization.

Indeed, evidence from the *Fourth National Survey of Ethnic Minorities* illustrates this point clearly. In that survey, analysis of ethnic differences in
income within class groups showed that, within each class group, ethnic
minority people had a lower income than white people (Nazroo, 2001).
Indeed, for the poorest group – Pakistani and Bangladeshi people – differences were twofold and equivalent in size to the difference between the
richest and poorest class groups in the white population. So the incomes
of Pakistani and Bangladeshi people in the richest class matched those of
white people in the poorest class, and, as the findings on income shown in
Table 2.1.3 suggest, there was little overlap in the income distributions of
these ethnic groups. And similar findings have been reported in the USA.
For example, there are racial differences in the quality of education, income returns for a given level of education or occupational status, wealth
or assets associated with a given level of income, the purchasing power
of income, the stability of employment, and the health risks associated
with occupational status (Williams and Collins, 1995). Similarly, Oliver
and Shapiro (1995) report that, within occupational groups, white people
have higher incomes than black people among those below the poverty
line. In addition, black people are more likely to remain in this situation
than white people, and, within income strata, black people have considerably lower wealth levels than white people and are less likely to be home
owners.

The overall conclusion, then, is that using single or crude indicators
of socio-economic position is of little use for 'controlling out' the impact of socio-economic position when attempting to reveal the extent
of a 'non-socio-economic' religion/ethnic/race effect. Within any given
level of a particular socio-economic indicator, the social circumstances
of the minority group is less favourable than those of the majority. This
leads to two related problems with approaches that attempt to adjust for
socio-economic effects when making comparisons across groups. The first
is that, if socio-economic position is simply regarded as a confounding
factor that needs to be controlled out to reveal the 'true' relationship
between religion/ethnicity and health, data will be presented and interpreted once controls have been applied. This will result in the impact
of socio-economic factors becoming obscured and their explanatory role
lost. The second is that the presentation of 'standardized' data allows the
problems with such data, outlined by Kaufman et al. (1998) and Nazroo

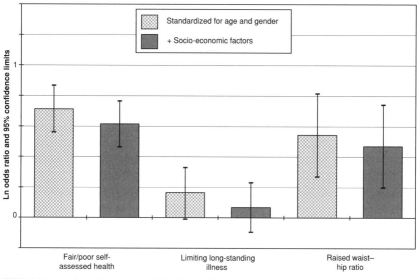

*White British and other white groups, excluding Irish people.

Figure 2.1.2 Socio-economic effects: Caribbean Christians compared with white Christians*

(2001), to be ignored, leaving both the author and reader to assume that all of any remaining 'ethnic/race' effect can be attributed to cultural or genetic factors. Nevertheless if these cautions are considered, there are some benefits in attempting to control for socio-economic effects. In particular, if controlling for socio-economic effects alters the pattern of ethnic inequalities in health, despite the limitations of the indicators used, we can conclude that at least a part of the differences we have uncovered are a result of a socio-economic effect.

We make some attempt to do that here. However, limited socio-economic measures in the HSE means that the analysis suffers from the problems just described, and small sample sizes mean that statistical power is poor and that the confidence intervals for coefficients in the models are large. Figures 2.1.2 and 2.1.3 show the contribution of socio-economic effects (economic activity, income, occupational class, highest educational qualification) to increased risks of health (fair/poor self-assessed health, limiting long-standing illness and raised waist–hip ratio) for two groups, Caribbean Christians and Muslims, compared with white Christians. Each bar shows the natural logarithm of the odds ratios and 95 per cent confidence intervals without and with socio-economic controls (natural logarithm is shown so that the visual size of the reduction is meaningful).

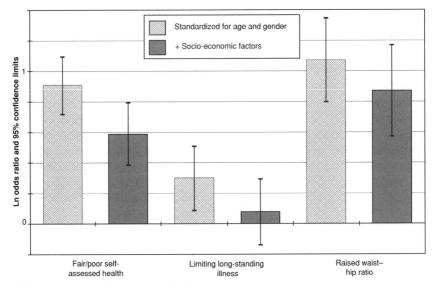

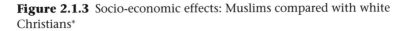
*White British and other white groups, excluding Irish people.

Figure 2.1.3 Socio-economic effects: Muslims compared with white Christians*

Although the analyses are limited, they indicate that socio-economic effects do contribute to the religious/ethnic inequalities in health observed in Table 2.1.2. In each case, the odds are reduced when socio-economic indicators are included in the model and, although differences remain significant, some of the reductions are large, particularly for the poorer Muslim groups.

Associations between health, racism and discrimination

The impact of racism on the health of minority groups is being increasingly recognized. Existing work has shown an impact on health for both the personal experience of racist victimization or discrimination, and fear of racism or belief that the majority population may be racist (for example, Karlsen and Nazroo, 2002, 2004; Krieger, 2000). However, while existing work shows that these effects persist across ethnic groups and contexts, they have not been examined in relation to religious minority groups. Here we use data from the *EMPIRIC* study to examine the relationship

Table 2.1.6 Risk of fair or poor self-assessed health with experiences and perceptions of discrimination

	Racial victimization in the past year	Believe half or more British employers discriminate	Either victimized or believe employers discriminate
	Age and gender standardized odds-ratio (95% C.I.) compared with those without experience of racism or belief of discrimination		
All minorities	1.70 (1.20,2.40)	1.52 (1.14,2.03)	1.63 (1.24,2.14)
Christian			
All	2.12 (1.15,3.93)	2.13 (1.34,3.39)	2.12 (1.33,3.38)
Irish	1.61 (0.61,4.24)	2.78 (1.36,5.68)	2.27 (1.12,4.59)
Non-white	3.27 (1.85,5.78)	1.78 (1.11,2.84)	2.20 (1.45,3.34)
No religion	1.61 (0.61,4.24)	1.71 (0.46,6.32)	2.04 (0.58,7.17)
Muslim	1.17 (0.74,1.86)	1.25 (0.77,2.03)	1.31 (0.85,2.02)
Sikh	1.52 (0.69,3.32)	0.68 (0.33,1.39)	1.02 (0.54,1.92)
Hindu	2.36 (0.85,6.55)	1.21 (0.61,2.38)	1.49 (0.81,2.74)

between experiences of racism and perceptions of discrimination and three health outcomes – self-assessed health, limiting long-standing illness and a common mental disorder – for the limited set of religious/ethnic categories that the *EMPIRIC* sample design allows. Findings for self-assessed health are shown in Table 2.1.6. The first row, which combines all of the religious/ethnic minority respondents, shows a clear effect for both of the measures we used (experience of racial victimization and belief that employers discriminate), and for when these measures are combined into a single index (the final column of the table). These effects are also apparent for both of the Christian minority groups, although they are not significant for Irish Christians and experience of racial victimization in the past year. They also appear to be present for the other religious minority groups, although none of the findings are statistically significant and some have an odds ratio that is either close to 1 or below 1.

Table 2.1.7 shows findings for reporting a limiting long-standing illness, which largely echo those for self-assessed health, although they are smaller and they are non-significant for non-white Christians. Table 2.1.8 shows findings for common mental disorder, and again these echo findings for the other two health outcomes, although the size of the effects is generally larger and more are statistically significant. It is worth noting that all three tables suggest that effects are similar for all of the religious minority

Table 2.1.7   Risk of limiting long-standing illness with experiences and perceptions of discrimination

	Racial victimization in the past year	Believe half or more British employers discriminate	Either victimized or believe employers discriminate
	Age and gender standardized odds-ratio (95% C.I.) compared with those without experience of racism or belief of discrimination		
All minorities	1.55 (1.04,2.29)	1.64 (1.19,2.26)	1.68 (1.25,2.26)
Christian			
All	1.85 (1.02,3.36)	2.25 (1.36,3.70)	2.19 (1.38,3.47)
Irish	1.89 (0.75,4.78)	3.91 (1.76,8.71)	3.29 (1.61,6.71)
Non-white	1.82 (1.04,3.19)	1.19 (0.76,1.87)	1.20 (0.77,1.86)
No religion	1.64 (0.44,6.05)	1.24 (0.54,2.83)	1.59 (0.69,3.68)
Muslim	1.28 (0.71,2.33)	1.30 (0.84,2.03)	1.31 (0.87,1.99)
Sikh	1.04 (0.32,3.42)	0.65 (0.26,1.67)	0.79 (0.34,1.83)
Hindu	1.90 (0.70,5.17)	1.47 (0.70,3.11)	1.84 (0.86,3.94)

Table 2.1.8   Risk of common mental disorder with experiences and perceptions of discrimination

	Racial victimization in the past year	Believe half or more British employers discriminate	Either victimized or believe employers discriminate
	Age and gender standardized odds-ratio (95% C.I.) compared with those without experience of racism or belief of discrimination		
All minorities	2.27 (1.61,3.19)	1.86 (1.377,2.53)	2.20 (1.66,2.92)
Christian			
All	2.64 (1.49,4.68)	2.08 (1.29,3.34)	2.44 (1.54,3.86)
Irish	2.53 (1.04,6.17)	2.44 (1.11,5.39)	2.64 (1.28,5.42)
Non-white	2.76 (1.56,4.90)	1.88 (1.22,2.91)	2.41 (1.53,3.80)
No religion	0.95 (0.28,3.17)	2.49 (0.81,7.64)	2.50 (0.75,8.34)
Muslim	1.88 (1.04,3.37)	1.63 (1.03,2.59)	1.93 (1.24,3.01)
Sikh	4.38 (1.93,9.94)	0.59 (0.22,1.58)	1.56 (0.74,3.32)
Hindu	3.24 (1.33,7.90)	1.77 (0.82,3.81)	1.87 (0.93,3.78)

groups, with the possible exception of Sikhs, for whom they may be a little smaller.

Conclusion

Although ethnic/race inequalities in health have been extensively studied, there has been little investigation of the patterning of health by religious identity. In this chapter, we have set out to begin to address this gap. Our analysis of data from the *Health Survey of England* (HSE) shows clear inequalities in health across religious groups, but also inequalities by ethnic category within religious groups. Inequalities across religious groups were most apparent for Muslim and Sikh people, while inequalities within religious groups were most apparent for Caribbean people. For 4 of the 5 health outcomes considered (self-assessed health, limiting long-standing illness, diabetes, and raised waist–hip ratio), Muslim people had markedly worse health than white Christians. Sikh people had an increased risk compared with the white Christian group for each of the five health outcomes, while Caribbean Christians had an increased risk for four of the outcomes, with differences only marginally not significantly greater for the fifth (limiting long-standing illness). Caribbean people with no religion had poorer health on three of the outcomes. However of these groups, Muslims had the greatest risk of poor health. In contrast, the health of Hindus, Buddhists, Indian, Chinese, Black African and Irish Christians, and white British and Chinese people with no religion compared relatively favourably with that of white Christians. Of these groups, Black African and Indian Christians and Hindus had the worst health, while the Chinese Christian, Chinese no-religion, and Buddhist groups had the best health.

Such an analysis does no more than provide a description of inequalities in health, however, and, while such a description might be important for planning services, it does little to add to our understanding of the causes of such inequalities. Elsewhere one of us has argued that an analysis of coronary heart disease risk by religion simply allows discussion of 'Muslim heart disease' rather than 'South Asian heart disease' (Nazroo, 2001). Rather, it is important to understand the factors that lead to an association between a religious/ethnic identity and health inequality, to understand how and why religious/ethnic identities are related to the factors that drive health inequalities, and to use such information to provide an impetus to address the social inequalities that are attached to religious/ethnic identities. Our analysis has shown the depth of socio-economic inequalities faced by some religious/ethnic minorities. In particular, Muslim groups face very marked inequalities and those for Caribbean and Sikh people are also large (indeed, the figures for Caribbean and Sikh people would be shocking if they were not placed in the context of those for the Muslim groups). Addressing such inequalities cannot be done with a modest policy ambition, but addressing them is important, not least because of the implications for health inequalities. Here we have shown the significance of socio-economic inequalities for the health of religious minority groups, and a strong body of evidence has been produced to show their significance for ethnic/race inequalities in health (see Nazroo and Williams, 2005, for an overview).

However, a consideration of socio-economic inequalities needs to move beyond the economic to also consider the social. Here we have examined experiences of racism and discrimination, and perceptions of living in a racist society (the belief that employers discriminate against minority groups) and have shown that these too relate to health outcomes for religious minority groups. This connects with the growing evidence on the significance of experiences of racism for the health of ethnic/racial minority groups and indicates the need to consider how religious identities, as well as ethnic and racial identities, become racialized. Indeed, we need to consider the ways in which stereotypes that draw on notions of race, ethnicity and religion (often at the same time) are mobilized to produce and justify the marginalization of minority groups. Here we suggest that the interest should not be on religion (or ethnicity) per se, but on how these social identities are racialised and the inequalities that are associated with them. It is also important, however, to consider the ways in which such identities may operate as a site of support and resistance (Solomos, 1998).

Acknowledgements

Work for this chapter was funded by the Economic and Social Research Council grant 'Being a Muslim in Europe: attitudes and experiences' (RES-163-25-0009).

References

Erens, B., Primatesta, P. and Prior, G. (2001) *Health Survey for England 1999: The Health of Minority Ethnic Groups*. London: The Stationery Office.

Harris, R., Tobias, M., Jeffreys, M. et al. (2006) Māori health and inequalities in New Zealand: the impact of racism and deprivation, *The Lancet*, 367: 2005–9.

Karlsen, S. and Nazroo, J.Y. (2000) Identity and structure: rethinking ethnic inequalities in health, in H. Graham (ed.) *Understanding Health Inequalities*. Buckingham: Open University Press.

Karlsen, S. and Nazroo, J.Y. (2002) The relationship between racial discrimination, social class and health among ethnic minority groups, *American Journal of Public Health*, 92(4): 624–31.

Karlsen, S. and Nazroo, J.Y. (2004) Fear of racism and health, *Journal of Epidemiology and Community Health*, 58(12): 1017–18.

Kaufman, J.S., Long, A.E., Liao, Y., Cooper, R.S. and McGee, D.L. (1998) The relation between income and mortality in U.S. blacks and whites, *Epidemiology*, 9(2): 147–55.

Krieger, N. (2000) Discrimination and health, in L. Berkman and I. Kawachi (eds) *Social Epidemiology*. Oxford: Oxford University Press.

Lewis, G., Pelosi, A.J., Araya, R.C. and Dunn, G. (1992) Measuring psychiatric disorder in the community: a standard assessment for use by lay interviewers, *Psychological Medicine*, 22: 465–86.

McLennan, W. and Madden, R. (1999) *The Health and Welfare of Australia's Aboriginal and Torres Strait Islander Peoples*. Commonwealth of Australia: Australian Bureau of Statistics.

Molarius, A. and Seidell, J.C. (1998) Selection of anthropometric indicators for classification of abdominal fatness: a critical review, *International Journal of Obesity*, 22: 719–27.

Nazroo, J.Y. (2001) *Ethnicity, Class and Health*. London: Policy Studies Institute.

Nazroo, J.Y. (2003) The structuring of ethnic inequalities in health: economic position, racial discrimination and racism, *American Journal of Public Health*, 93(2): 277–84.

Nazroo, J.Y., and Williams, D.R. (2005) The social determination of ethnic/racial inequalities in health, in M. Marmot and R.G. Wilkinson (eds) *Social Determinants of Health*. Oxford: Oxford University Press.

Oliver, M.L. and Shapiro, T.M. (1995) *Black Wealth/White Wealth: A New Perspective on Racial Inequality*. New York: Routledge.

Pan American Health Organization (2001) *Equity in Health: From an Ethnic Perspective*. Washington DC: Pan American Health Organization.

Sidiropoulos, E., Jeffery, A., Mackay, S. et al. (1997) *South Africa Survey 1996/97*. Johannesburg: South African Institute of Race Relations.

Smith, P. and Prior, G. (1997) *The Fourth National Survey of Ethnic Minorities: Technical Report*. London: Social and Community Planning Research.

Solomos, J. (1998) Beyond racism and multiculturalism, *Patterns of Prejudice*, 32(4): 45–62.

Sproston, K. and Mindell, J. (2006) *Health Survey for England 2004: The Health of Minority Ethnic Groups*. London: National Centre for Social Research.

Sproston, K. and Nazroo, J. (2002) *Ethnic Minority Psychiatric Illness Rates in the Community (EMPIRIC.)* London: The Stationery Office.

Williams, D.R. (2001) Racial variations in adult health status: Patterns, paradoxes and prospects, in N. Smelser, W.J. Wilson and F. Mitchell (eds) *America Becoming: Racial Trends and Their Consequences, National Research Council Commission on Behavioral and Social Sciences and Education*. Washington DC: National Academy of Sciences Press.

Williams, D.R. and Collins, C. (1995) U.S. socioeconomic and racial differences in health: patterns and explanations, *Annual Review of Sociology*, 21: 349–86.

2.2 Negotiating ethnic identities and health

Karl Atkin

Introduction

Public health research and policy in the UK, as in other high-income countries, have long been concerned with social inequalities in health. However, the concern has taken a particular form. Rather than an engagement with how multiple dimensions of social inequality impact on people's health across the population, the focus is often on one specific dimension of social inequality. In addition, it has been socio-economic inequalities among 'white' men which have attracted most research interest and policy attention. Only recently has UK research and policy begun to recognize ethnicity as a dimension of social inequality with implications for people's health. For the 'white' population, however, ethnicity is rarely discussed as a dimension of people's identity; and is rarely seen to offer any insights into their experiences of health. For non-white populations, ethnicity is almost always noted and tends to be seen as dominating all other aspects of a person's identity. In these populations, ethnicity is seen to capture the 'essence' of who the person is and therefore the primary determinant of their health (Karlsen and Nazroo, 2006). Ethnicity is thus represented as both fixed and homogenous; as having the same meaning in all contexts for everyone who is defined as a member of that minority ethnic group (Ahmad and Bradby, 2007).

This essentializing view of ethnicity has been repeatedly challenged (see Atkin and Chattoo, 2007). It has been pointed out that not every aspect of a person's identity and experience – and not every aspect of their health and encounters with the health care system – can be explained by his or her ethnic background. As among the 'white' population, a person's identity, like their health experiences and health care encounters, will be influenced by their age, gender and socio-economic position, as well as by how others respond to these different dimensions of identity. Because these multiple influences on identity can be hard to capture in quantitative studies of health, researchers have looked to qualitative approaches to enable people to talk about when and how ethnicity makes a difference – and when it does not.

The chapter contributes to this more nuanced approach to ethnic identity and health. It discusses – by way of context – how health researchers have engaged with ethnicity and the theoretical debates which are changing how they understand it. The chapter then introduces two qualitative studies. The first focused on young people who could be broadly classified as being of 'South Asian' origin and who are hearing-impaired. It explored their wish to express their Deaf identities while also celebrating their cultural and ethnic identities (the use of a capital 'D' is also explained). The second involved members of different ethnic minority groups at risk of haemoglobin disorders, and explored how religion and faith influenced decisions about antenatal screening for sickle cell and thalassaemia disorders. The chapter ends by reflecting on the implications of the studies for advancing understandings of ethnic identity within health research and health policy.

Understanding ethnic identity

Identity is a field of research in many academic disciplines, including psychology, sociology and philosophy. The result is a wide array of perspectives, with rich debates within and between them (Jenkins, 2004). Across these perspectives, however, there is some important common ground.

There is a broad agreement that identity is an awareness of who one is and where one belongs. It is widely agreed, too, that identity is both self-determined and shaped by the definitions of others. On the one hand, it is an expression of individual agency, offering a mobilizing resource which enables people to realize and celebrate who they are. On the other, it is constantly subject to negotiation, both within personal networks of family, friends and communities and within impersonal structures – the school, the workplace, the welfare state – which regulate people's lives. These social institutions can both facilitate and constrain the expression of identity, with some groups having more space and opportunity to realize their sense of identity than others. A member of a minority ethnic group, for example, may experience their time at school or in the workplace as an ongoing struggle to negotiate and express an identity which is true to the individual's own cultural and religious identifications. As this suggests, issues of power are intimately bound up with identity and the extent to which the expression of identity is the outcome of individual agency or constrained by social structure. Building on this, there is a broad measure of agreement that identity is dynamic, not fixed (Giddens, 1991). Not only does our sense of who we are and where we belong change as we grow up, it also changes across the different contexts of our lives. Our sense of identity is likely to be different at home than it is beyond it; and to be different at school and in the workplace than in a place of worship.

Running across debates about identity is an appreciation that it is always multiple: who we are and where we belong has many aspects (see Du Gay et al., 2000). Most of the leading theorists on identity agree that each individual combines different identities: for example, in the context of our case studies, a familial identity (daughter, mother), a religious identity, an identity as a young person and an identity as an individual with disabilities. There is likely to be a constant interplay between these different aspects of identity, with some experienced as more important and more supported (or more under threat) in some contexts than in others (see Lawler, 2008).

As this brief summary suggests, a series of common themes run through contemporary debates about identity. These emphasize that an individual's sense of who they are is part of a constant negotiation between agency and structure, it is influenced by context, and it is multiple and shifting.

When it comes to ethnic identity however, much health research and policy and much health care practice seems to draw on a different set of assumptions (Ahmad and Bradby, 2007). Differences between dominant and minority cultures tend to be over-emphasized, with the result that ethnicity is assumed to dominate all aspects of identity for those identified as belonging to a minority culture (Chattoo and Ahmad, 2008). For example, it is often assumed that any and all difficulties that the individual faces – including with respect to their health and to the health care system – can be attributed to his or her ethnic background. While challenged by research, such assumptions are in accord with those found among the public at large (Kymlicka, 2001). The assumption that ethnicity is the dominant identity for members of minority ethnic groups is fundamental to the way in which ethnicity is 'imagined' in post-industrial societies like the UK (see, for example, accounts of 'ethnicity and culture' in most NHS National Service Frameworks). This way of representing ethnicity turns it from one dimension of who someone is into the whole of who they are: it 'essentializes' ethnicity. As Ahmad (1996: 32) notes, when it is stripped of its dynamic quality and isolated from its context, 'culture – and its expression through ethnicity – becomes a rigid constraint concept, which is seen to mechanically determine people's behaviours and actions rather than proving a flexible resource for living, and according meaning to what one feels, experiences and acts to change'. Further, once ethnicity is cast as the essence of identity, it is only a short step to social stereotypes which are seen to have explanatory value (Atkin and Chattoo, 2007).

The task for those working in health research and policy is to challenge this limited view of ethnic identity and to open up these fields to more nuanced understandings of ethnicity (Phillips, 2007). Like identity in general, ethnic identity is actively negotiated within the context of people's everyday social relationships and through their interactions with state institutions like the school, the National Health Service and the social security system (see Taylor, 1994). Like identity in general, it is also multi-faceted (Bradby, 2003). As a result, ethnicity is more than simply 'being of' or 'belonging to' an ethnic group but is an expression of a person's negotiation of multiple identities within different social and historical contexts (Atkin and Chattoo, 2007). Seen in this way, ethnic identity is complex and shifting, reflecting an ongoing dialogue between culture, ancestry, histories of migration, language, faith and religion, nationality and a shared heritage (Modood et al., 1997). Different aspects of ethnic identity can, in equal measure, support, sustain, reinforce and contradict each other (Hall, 1996). As we shall see, ethnicity and religious identity often inform each other, especially for people of South Asian origin (for a broader discussion, see Keay, 2000). At the same time, other aspects of a person's identity can intercede in the process, aspects which others can mistakenly attribute to ethnicity (Karslen and Nazroo, 2006).

Studies highlighting the contribution of socio-economic factors challenge assumptions that the poor health of some ethnic groups is explained by attributes of ethnicity (and cultural practices). As Nazroo's (1997) work demonstrates, socio-economic inequalities between ethnic groups are a primary cause of health inequalities between ethnic groups. As another example, South Asian and African-Caribbean women can struggle to convince doctors that their children are seriously ill and find themselves being dismissed as 'neurotic' or 'over-protective' (Anionwu and Atkin, 2001). Such views become explained by a lack of language support, assumptions about the passivity of South Asian women, along with patronizing attitudes about African-Caribbean women's ability to understand what they are being told. Nonetheless, a woman's treatment is not wholly a consequence of her ethnic background, but can be explained by doctors' more general sexist attitudes, which means they do not take mothers' views seriously (Green and Murton, 1996).

Other examples may help to ground the complex debates about ethnic identity in the lives of people of ethnic minority origin. A focus on young people's lives can help to do this. It is widely appreciated that young people born and brought up in the UK have different experiences and expectations from their parents, who may still perceive themselves, metaphorically at least, as 'immigrants' (Ali, 2003). But as this 15-year-old girl of Pakistani origin notes, the claims of young people to be 'British' can remain contingent: 'You say you're British, you *are* British...but then again, you know, in some people's eyes you're Asian

British, not *British* British' (Atkin and Chattoo, 2007: 387). Even so, young people of African-Caribbean origin are more likely to favour the label of 'Black' British or British-Caribbean than their parents and grandparents (Modood et al., 1997). Young people of South Asian origin, on the other hand, are increasingly using religious affiliations, such as Muslim or Hindu or Sikh, in addition to ethnic origin, when describing their identity, hence the popularity of terms such as British Muslim (Ahmad and Bradby, 2007). This is why, for some Pakistani and Bangladeshi Muslims living in the UK, religion can represent more than an expression of personal faith and also be a political statement (Craig, 2007). Their sense of Britishness is an expression of their citizenship claims within the context of a political environment which is increasingly ambivalent about such claims, while their faith identification marks out and celebrates their 'difference'.

In the process of articulating the more creative aspects of who they are, young people often begin to rethink their parents' identities (Anthias, 2002). African-Caribbean young people, when discussing their reproductive options, are likely to describe their parents' values as 'traditional' and at times, 'inflexible' (see Atkin et al., 2008). Some Muslim young people whose families originate from the Punjab criticize their parents' interpretation of Islam as embodying cultural practices which have nothing to do with faith (Atkin and Chattoo, 2007). Their parents, for their part, express concerns that their children's ethnic and broader cultural values are becoming corrupted by Western practices. However, the evidence points to considerable continuity in values between the different generations (Modood et al., 1997). Young people, although expressing their identity in relation to their broader engagement with British society in ways which might be different from their parents, do not wholly reject their parents' identifications (Bauman, 1996). Ethnic and cultural identity is still an important way of life for young people of ethnic minority origin (see Brah, 2006). Muslim young women, for example, rarely question the need to maintain modesty as a way of protecting their gendered moral integrity, but disagree when their parents suggest it can only be maintained with culturally specific dress associated with their families' countries of origin (Hussain et al., 2002).

There is, however, another dimension informing the process of rethinking identity. In defining who they are, both parents and their offspring can present themselves as an 'imagined' moral community. Identity can sometimes be represented as an attempt to restore the purity and recover the unity of previously imagined ethnic identities, which are felt to be lost as a response to coming to terms with new cultures around them (Hall, 1996). In the UK, this process has been linked, at least in part, to experiences of social exclusion and racism among minority ethnic populations (Ratcliffe, 2004). However, the assertion of a unifying ethnic identity can involve homogenizing difference and celebrating uniqueness, which in turn can reinforce dominant stereotypes (see Anderson, 2006).

Negotiating identities: Deafness and ethnic identity

The chapter now turns to the first of two case studies to explore how people negotiate their ethnicity within the context of their health. This concerns the intersections between deaf and ethnic identities.

Over the last two decades, understandings of deafness and other impairments have been transformed by what is called 'the social model of disability'. This powerful critique argues that many of the disadvantages faced by people with impairments result from the barriers that society places in their way, including discriminatory policies, for example around education and employment (Swain et al., 2004). With respect to deafness, systematic discrimination not only leads to loss of independence and choice, but also excludes deaf people from roles taken for granted by the majority of the population (Corker and French, 1999). Inclusion and claims to equal citizenship emerge as important symbols in the positive reframing of Deafness (Corker, 2002). This is reflected in a discursive strategy, in which those who ascribe to a more political identity refer to themselves as *Deaf* (with the emphasis on the capital D), rather than *deaf*. The chapter respects this convention.

Despite its value, a more social model of Deafness has tended, until recently, to give little consideration to diversity, particularly in relation to ethnic, cultural or religious identity (Ahmad et al., 1998; Chamba et al., 1998). Deaf culture seems predisposed to prioritize Deaf identity as the primary identity, emphasizing the shared oppression of Deaf people by a hearing society and a unity in values and language, such as the use of British Sign Language (BSL). If considered at all, diversity is seen as a potential threat, diluting claims of equality (see Ahmad et al., 2001). Further tensions emerge over the extent to which the social model assumes Eurocentric values (see Islam, 2008).

Exploring this potential tension represents the core theme of our first case study: a project funded by the UK's Economic and Social Research Council (see Ahmad et al., 2002; Atkin et al., 2002; Jones et al., 2002). It involved in-depth interviews with 25 young people, aged between 14 and 27 years, who could broadly be classified as being of 'South Asian' origin. These included 16 young people who described themselves as Pakistani Muslim, five as Indian Hindu, three as Indian Sikh and one as Indian Muslim (from East Africa). We also spoke to 15 family members who assumed parental responsibility for the deaf young person, and this sample included ten mothers, three fathers, one aunt and one sister. Eleven of this sample of family members described themselves as Pakistani Muslim, two as Indian Hindu, one as Indian Sikh and one as Indian Muslim from East Africa. All names in this and the other case study are pseudonyms.

The young people in the study made clear that they wished to express their sense of Deafness, while also celebrating their cultural and ethnic diversity. They wanted to do this, too, in the context of being a young person and through the symbols associated with youth culture. However, at the same time, restrictive disability and racist discourses constrained and denied them opportunities for expressing their chosen identities. Young people often associated with a Deaf identity, to the extent that they regarded it as offering the potential for empowerment. Interestingly, however, this cultural identity was also realized within the context of being 'British', which for some young people was seen to offer more 'respect' to deaf people than say Pakistani or Indian contexts. 'Britishness', therefore, assumed a positive connotation, which occurred simultaneously with a more negative association, acquired in relation to racist discursive practices and their sense of not being *British* British (see above).

Young people needed both an environment and resources to articulate a Deaf identity. This might include access to BSL as well as social networks which included other Deaf people. Without these resources, young people struggled to conceptualize their deafness as positive; with them, Deaf identity became potentially reaffirming. Twenty-year-old Sadhna Patel reflected on her contact with deaf people: '[They] helped build me up, if you like, make me feel positive, one step at the time. I had to think how to become strong. I've learnt to develop myself'.

Young people explained how Deaf identity made them feel 'normal' although, interestingly, this could also be seen as a means of giving young people more generic access to 'youth culture', independent of Deaf identity *per se*. 'Being' a young person represented an important aspect of how someone with Deafness saw him/herself. Some young women and men, for example, realized this through their interest in music, and wearing smart and fashionable clothes. This, however, was not about being 'Westernised'. Many talked about Indian films, Asian satellite television, Asian fashion magazines, as an expression of 'cool' and 'fashionable', reflecting the more general interests of their hearing peers.

Nonetheless, sustaining a Deaf identity was far from straightforward. To begin with, hearing family members regarded Deaf Culture with some ambivalence. The teaching of BSL and encouraging contacts with other

Deaf young people, either through schools or social networks, sometimes frustrated parents, who felt it contributed to their children's lack of ethnic and cultural capital. Parents expressed particular concerns over their ability to protect a young person's moral, cultural and religious identity. This perhaps is best summed up by a mother's comment: 'I send my son to school and he comes back an Englishman'. Parents expressed particular concerns about 'losing their child'. Some, for example, saw the exclusive imposition of BSL at the expense of more multi-lingual strategies as undermining their relationships with their children and, more broadly, as a means of imposing Eurocentric values and assumptions. To this extent, parents perceived any threat to 'home' language as a symbolic threat to community relationships, cultural reproduction and religious practice. Kaneez Rasool, whose 17-year-old son had learnt BSL, commented, 'They understood us more when they were little. Now they have their *own* language, not just *our way* of communicating'.

Young people, on the other hand, felt that parents failed to see the positive aspects of Deaf identity and, despite describing loving family relationships, some said they were isolated and under-valued in their families. Fifteen-year-old Bushra Khan, for example, was aware that her parents struggled with having a deaf child and, although she knew they loved her, felt that they had little confidence in her abilities: '[My mother] was upset...she wanted me hearing like everyone else. She did not want a deaf child.'

Young people specifically felt their parents' views of deafness undermined their own confidence and particularly reflected on how their parents' low expectations made it more difficult for them to realize their potential in relation to education, social life and work. John Kang, aged 12, said, 'My father is not aware of what deaf people are capable of. He does not think we can do anything at all.' Bushra described her parents' surprise when they discovered she could learn English. She was upset, however at how her parents continued to treat her hearing siblings more favourably. This treatment was seen to subvert 'normal' family hierarchies in a way evident in other young people's accounts: 'It seems as though, because I am deaf, they kept me in the background. They always involved my younger sister. I think it is because I am deaf. They don't think I can handle things.'

Young people, however, did not seek to reject their parents' cultural or religious values, although they did recognize their Deafness made it difficult for them to realize them. Most, for example, ranked their religious identity as one of the most important aspects of who they were, although the same people ranked 'Deafness' equally high, suggesting both are important to young people's perceptions of who they are. Problems in communicating with their parents meant they did not always have the same access to religious or cultural socialization as their hearing peers. This was also reflected in broader community networks. Mosques and temples, for example, rarely engaged with a young person's communication needs. Twenty-two-year-old Adeeba Ahmad remarked, 'I don't know anything about Islam. I have no idea about it. I never went to Mosque . . . I know we eat halal meat, but I do not know what it is.'

A deaf young person's limited understanding of religion, both in terms of scripture and values, concerned parents greatly. Despite this, most young people felt they knew enough about religious and cultural values, perhaps reflecting their importance to them. Indeed, the narratives of deaf young people of South Asian origin suggested they were able to challenge their parents' religious values as being an expression of cultural norms, in the same way as their peers (see above). Seventeen-year-old Misbah Nabi's comments reflected this: 'My mother says clothes, like skirts and tops, mother says I am not allowed to wear that. I think that is strange, because it's all right. It's long, so my mother is wrong. As long as you are covered up, it's OK.'

Broader tensions also emerged during this process of cultural reconstitution. Shehnaz Akhter wanted to meet other Deaf people, but acknowledged that her mother was concerned about 'mixing with boys'. Several other young people expressed similar awareness of, and frustration at, potential tensions between Deaf culture and their own wish to express a distinct cultural identity. They did not see the two as incompatible.

Nonetheless, a few young people were attracted to 'white' Deaf culture and the freedoms it offered. The problems of religious and cultural socialization made this an option for them, in a way that it might not be for their hearing peers, although it tended to be only available to young men, providing further evidence for the multi-faceted way in which identity is negotiated. Parents, as we have seen, felt deafness made their children vulnerable and often responded differently to young men and women because of the gendered nature of moral identities (see also Katbamna et al., 2000).

To summarize, the accounts of these young people provide little support for notions of a singular or primary identity which made other identity claims irrelevant. Most wished to combine a positive self-identity with the need to live within specific cultural and religious contexts. Deaf culture offered many advantages to a young person but it sometimes failed to recognize and provide for cultural or religious sensitivities. Negotiating this remained fundamental to a young person's sense of identity and it was rare for young people to feel they could only be 'one thing'. In cultivating and legitimating identities, however, tensions reflecting broader power relationships emerged. Not only was a young person actively creating a positive identity, they were doing so within a context that attempted to impose choices (and disadvantages) on them, which might or might not reflect their sense of who they were.

Negotiating identities: faith, prenatal diagnosis and termination

Our second case-study comes from a project involving ethnic minority groups at risk of haemoglobin disorders (Ahmed et al., 2006; Atkin et al., 2008). Again, the study employed a qualitative methodology, but this time involved focus groups with men and women from a variety of 'faith' communities (Muslim, Sikh, Hindu and Christian) and different ethnic minority groups (Pakistani, Indian and African-Caribbean). The fieldwork had two phases. One set of focus groups involved people of reproductive age talking about the influence of faith in making reproductive decisions; the other involved community and religious representatives, and explored their potential role in influencing people's decision making.

The study was funded by England's National Screening Committee for Sickle Cell and Thalassaemia Disorders, a government-appointed committee with responsibility for determining screening policies and procedures. The study's aim was to help inform an effective screening programme for women whose pregnancies are 'at risk' of a sickle cell or thalassaemia disorder. As such, the questions it was designed to answer reflected how ethnicity, and faith in particular, was imagined by the policy-making community. The screening programme involves offering prenatal diagnosis for sickle cell or thalassaemia disorders to women and their partners, with those diagnosed at risk presented with the option of either continuing or terminating the pregnancy. This, however, involves difficult and complex choices, in which couples not only draw on their understanding of sickle cell and thalassaemia but also broader aspects of their identity. A person's faith might be a factor when exploring decision making, as either a reason for declining prenatal diagnosis and termination of pregnancy (Rozario, 2005) or for providing a public context in which decisions take place (Shaw, 2000).

Despite such assumptions informing the initial policies of the National Screening Committee on Sickle Cell and Thalassaemia Disorders, the commissioned research contradicted them. We found that decision making about prenatal diagnosis was multi-faceted, with religious belief more important to some people than others (see also Tsianakas and Liamputtong, 2002). Further, religious identity among our participants was not something pre-defined, but was produced and negotiated within a particular social context and in relation to the values of significant others (see also Inhorn, 2006). There appeared to be no particular script pre-defining how religious norms and practices would mediate the decision-making process.

Faith beliefs emerged as flexible, negotiable and contingent: a resource which could be used creatively to support and legitimate a person's decision. Beliefs were rarely seen as prescriptive – as providing a rigid sense of right and wrong – but were seen as part of a broader moral framework (see also Kleinman, 2006).

In the first set of focus groups, participants – irrespective of faith – emphasized that, although taking a life through termination of pregnancy might be regarded as 'a sin', this had to be balanced against 'preventing suffering', which required individual interpretation. According to the participants, this is why God gave people free-will. As one Hindu man observed, 'if there is no free-will, there is no need for God'. A Pakistani Muslim man explained further: 'We are not like robots. We can make our own decision. He (God) has shown us the right path and the wrong path and he says we can make our own decision.' An African-Caribbean Christian woman agreed: 'Follow the spirit of God and he will guide you and lead you because no one is perfect in life.' As part of this, people see responsibilities for their own future, as well as family and personal relationships, as equally influential when making a decision to seek prenatal diagnosis (see also Remennick, 2006). Previous experience of the condition and judgments about its severity also assumed significance during the decision-making process, in addition to reflections on how the broader society treated people with chronic illness and disability. Religious beliefs are not regarded as offering an absolute moral code but more of a framework in which to make decisions. People's interpretation of *fatwas* demonstrates this further.

Some Islamic States have *fatwas*, permitting the termination of pregnancy before 120 days of gestation following a prenatal diagnosis of thalassaemia (see Abdel Haleem, 1993). Muslim participants, however, still interpreted *fatwas* within the context of their own beliefs and experiences. Some welcomed *fatwas* in helping them come to a decision about prenatal diagnosis, while others stated that they would not consider termination as an option because of their own moral beliefs. Some participants also pointed out that, since they had been produced in places such as Lebanon, Saudi Arabia and Pakistan, they might not be applicable to Western countries, where the more ready availability of treatment made children less likely to suffer.

People of all faiths, although acknowledging a potential role for religious representatives, remained ambivalent about consulting them regarding prenatal diagnosis. People were especially concerned that advice from religious representatives might be too prescriptive. However, in the second set of focus groups with religious representatives, they made it clear – irrespective of faith – that they did not see their role as prescribing beliefs or behaviour. Instead, religious belief was perceived as a personal matter, between an individual and God. Representatives emphasized that their role was to support people rather than tell them what to do. The onus was on the individual to make a decision, which they could justify and with which they could live.

Faith representatives expressed more general concerns about the involvement of religious leaders in what they regarded as health matters. Hindu religious representatives, for example, felt they had no role in offering advice on health matters: 'We shouldn't be training religious leaders on health issues. It's just being politically correct. If there is just the sense that a religious leader has been included then that's ok.' Representatives pointed out that raising community awareness in minority ethnic groups should not be seen as different from the process for raising awareness in the 'white' community. The faith workshops were especially concerned that a reliance on religious and community leaders could absolve the British State of a more meaningful engagement with ethnic minority populations. A participant in the African-Caribbean Christian workshop said, 'It's convenient to speak to one person or a small group of people and then it appears as if they have communicated to the masses.' This suggests a potential flaw in government policies which assume that 'faith' offers a way of engaging with ethnic minority populations. Religious conviction was important in explaining people's attitudes to prenatal diagnosis but it was not the only influence. Individuals, therefore, were not a straightforward embodiment of their faith. Engaging with them as such ran the risk of institutionalizing an essentialized notion of ethnicity within the screening programme which reflected wider stereotypes rather than a person's sense of who they were.

Conclusion

This chapter engages with how ethnic identity is produced within particular social contexts associated with health. It suggests that ethnic identity is not fixed or predefined, but will have different meanings both for different people and for the same individual in different situations. In some instances, a person may wish to emphasize their religious identity; in others, their sense of national heritage might be important. At other times, it might be their deafness or gender. Equally, expressing one aspect of their identity at expense of another rarely reflects the way people live their lives. For example, people might wish to celebrate their Deaf identity, while also taking pride in being Muslim or Hindu.

This is why the chapter challenges the idea of essentialized identities and suggests, instead, that there are no singular identities or hierarchies of identification with which policy and practice can engage. A person rarely sees themselves wholly as being deaf or their membership of a particular faith community as defining everything about them. Instead, they negotiate and realize their identity within the context of other aspects of their life. The presumption that there is one aspect of a person's identity, in which all other expressions must be reflected, fails to capture the complexity of who we are.

Further, the chapter has noted how others may challenge a person's definitions of self-identity, seeking to impose their own. Thus, individual interpretation becomes embedded in a conditional acceptance derived from and sustained by the social relationships which surround them. Attempts by individuals, whether they have deafness or are at risk of a genetic condition, to define themselves will also be influenced by major social institutions, including the health service. Institutions representing the state tend to engage with people as conglomerates and stereotypes, emphasizing certain essentialized aspects of their disability, gender, social class, cultural, religion or ethnic group, rather than as citizens with multiple identities (Das, 1995). This suggests that the policy and practice communities need to question how they define and 'imagine' ethnicity (and disability, gender and social class too) in a way that enables them to respond to the needs of people from minority ethnic populations without recourse to generalized notions of culture or community (see Parekh, 2002). Successful interventions catering for a diverse population are ones which do not rely on stereotyping the people to whom they deliver care (Papadopoulos et al., 2004). This requires that policy makers, service managers and practitioners are able to work with an individual's own definitions of who they are (see Atkin and Chattoo, 2007).

Acknowledgments

The Economic and Social Research Council funded the original research on Deafness (Project reference: 00237122). The Antenatal and Newborn Screening Programme (Sickle Cell and Thalassaemia) funded the research on faith and prenatal screening. I would like to thank Sangeeta Chattoo, who for many years now has been always willing to exchange ideas and engage in discussion, while also acknowledging a more distant but nonetheless significant intellectual debt to Waqar Ahmad, who made me think about ethnicity in an entirely different way. Valuable discussions with Hilary Graham also helped develop the text.

References

Abdel Haleem, M.A.S. (1993) Medical ethics in Islam, in A. Grubb (ed.) *Choices and Decisions in Health Care.* Chichester: John Wiley and Sons.

Ahmad, W.I.U. (1996) The trouble with culture, in D. Kellher and S. Hillier (eds) *Researching Cultural Differences in Health*. London: Routledge.

Ahmad, W.I.U. and Bradby, H. (2007) Locating ethnicity and health: exploring concepts and contexts, *Sociology of Health and Illness*, 29(6): 793–811.

Ahmad, W.I.U., Atkin, K. and Jones, L. (2002) Being deaf and being other things: South Asian deaf young people and identity negotiation, *Social Science and Medicine*, 55(10): 1757–69.

Ahmad, W.I.U., Darr, A. and Jones, L. (2001) 'I send my child to school and he comes back an Englishman': minority ethnic deaf people, identity politics and services' in W.I.U. Ahmad (ed.) *Ethnicity, Disability and Chronic Illness*. Buckingham: Open University Press.

Ahmad, W.I.U., Darr, A., Jones, L. and Gohar, N. (1998) *Deafness and Ethnicity: Services, Policy and Politics*. Bristol: Policy Press.

Ahmed, S., Atkin, K., Hewison, J. and Green, J. (2006) The influence of faith and religion and the role of religious leaders in prenatal diagnosis for sickle cell disorders and thalassaemia major, *Prenatal Diagnosis*, 26: 801–9.

Ali, N. (2003) Diaspora and nation: displacement and the politics of Kashmiri identity in Britain, *Contemporary South Asia*, 12(4): 471–80.

Anderson, B. (2006) *Imagined Communities*. London: Verso.

Anionwu, E. and Atkin, K. (2001) *The Politics of Sickle Cell and Thalassaemia*. Buckingham: Open University Press.

Anthias, F. (2002) 'Where do I belong?': narrating collective identity and translocation positionality, *Ethnicities*, 2(4): 491–514.

Atkin, K. and Chattoo, S. (2007) The dilemmas of providing welfare in an ethnically diverse state: seeking reconciliation in the role of a 'reflexive practitioner', *Policy and Politics*, 35(3): 379–95.

Atkin, K., Ahmad, W.I.U. and Jones, L. (2002) Young Asian deaf people and their families: negotiating relationships and identities, *Sociology of Health and Illness*, 24(1): 21–45.

Atkin, K., Ahmed, S., Green, J. and Hewison, J. (2008) Decision making and ante-natal screening for sickle cell and thalassaemia disorders: to what extent do faith and religious identity mediate choice? *Current Sociology*, 56(1): 77–98.

Bauman, G. (1996) *Contesting Culture: Discourses of Identity in Multi-ethnic London*. Cambridge: Cambridge University Press.

Bradby, H. (2003) Describing ethnicity in health research, *Ethnicity and Health*, 8(1): 5–14.

Brah, A. (2006) 'The 'Asian' in Britain, in N. Ali, S. Karla and S. Sayyid (eds) *A Postcolonial People: South Asians in Britain*. London: Hurst.

Chamba, R., Ahmad, W. and Jones, L. (1998) *Improving Services for Asian Deaf Children: Patient and Professionals' Perspectives*. Bristol: Policy Press.

Chattoo, S. and Ahmad, W.I.U. (2008) The moral economy of selfhood and caring: negotiating boundaries of personal care as embodied moral practice, *Sociology of Health and Illness*, 30(4): 550–64.

Corker, M. (2002) Disability politics: language, planning and inclusion in social policy, *Disability and Society*, 15(3): 445–62.

Corker, M. and French, S. (1999) *Disability Discourse*. Buckingham: Open University Press.

Craig, G. (2007) Cunning, unprincipled, loathsome: the racist tail wags the welfare dog, *Journal of Social Policy*, 36(4): 605–23.

Das, V. (1995) *Critical Events: An Anthropological Perspective on Contemporary India*. Oxford: Oxford University Press.

Du Gay, P., Evans, J. and Redman, P. (2000) *Identity: A Reader*. London: SAGE.

Giddens, A. (1991) *Modernity and Self-identity: Self and Society in Late Modern Age*. Cambridge: Polity Press.

Green, J. and Murton, F.E. (1996) Diagnosis of Duchenne Muscular Dystrophy: parents' experiences and satisfaction, *Child Care, Health and Development*, 22(2): 113–28.

Hall, S. (1996) Introduction: who needs identity, in S. Hall and P. du Gay (eds) *Questions of Cultural Identity*. London: SAGE.

Hussain, Y., Atkin, K. and Ahmad, W.I.U. (2002) *South Asian Young People and Disability*. Bristol: Policy Press.

Islam, Z. (2008) Negotiating identities: the lives of Pakistani and Bangladeshi young disabled people, *Disability and Society*, 23(1): 41–52.

Inhorn, M.C. (2006) Making Muslim babies: IVF and gamete donation in Sunni versus Shi'a Islam, *Culture, Medicine and Psychiatry*, 30: 427–50.

Jenkins, R. (2004) *Social Identity*. London: Routledge.

Jones, L., Atkin, K. and Ahmad, W.I.U. (2002) Supporting Asian deaf young people and their families: the role of professionals and services, *Disability and Society*, 16(1): 51–70.

Karlsen, S. and Nazroo, J. (2006) Defining and measuring ethnicity and 'race': theoretical and conceptual issues for health and social care research, in J.Y. Nazroo, (ed.) *Health and social research in multiethnic societies*. London: Routledge.

Katbamna, S., Bhakta, P. and Parker, G. (2000) Perceptions of disability and care-giving relationships in South Asian communities, in W.I.U. Ahmad (ed.) *Ethnicity, Disability and Chronic Illness*. Buckingham: Open University Press.

Keay, J. (2000) *India: A History*. London: Harper Perennial.

Kleinman, A. (2006) *What Really Matters: Living a Moral Life amidst Uncertainty and Danger*. Oxford: Oxford University Press.

Kymlicka, W. (2001) *Politics in the Vernacular: Nationalism, Multiculturalism and Citizenship*. Oxford: Oxford University Press.

Lawler, S. (2008) *Identity: Sociological Perspectives*. Cambridge: Polity Press.

Modood, T., Betthould, R., Lakey, J. et al. (1997) *Ethnic Minorities in Britain*. London: Policy Studies Institute.

Nazroo, J. (1997) *The Health of Britain's Ethnic Minorities*. London: Policy Studies Institute.

Papadopoulos, I., Tilkim M. and Lees, S. (2004) Promoting cultural competence in health care through a research-based intervention in the UK, *Diversity in Health and Social Care*, 1(2): 107–16.

Parekh, B. (2006) *Rethinking Multiculturalism: Cultural Diversity and Political Theory*. Basingstoke: Macmillan.

Phillips, A. (2007) *Multi-culturalism without Culture*. Princeton, NJ: Princeton University Press.

Ratcliffe, P. (2004) *'Race', Ethnicity and Difference*. Maidenhead: Open University Press.

Remennick, L. (2006) The quest for the perfect baby: why do Israeli women seek prenatal genetic testing? *Sociology of Health and Illness*, 28(1): 21–53.

Rozario, S. (2005) Genetics, religion and identity among British Bangladeshis: some initial findings, *Diversity in Health and Social Care*, 2: 187–96.

Shaw, A. (2000) *Kinship and Continuity: Pakistani Families in Britain*. Singapore: Harwood.

Swain, J., Barnes, C., French, S. and Thomas, C. (2004) *Disabling Barriers, Enabling Environments*. London: SAGE.

Taylor, C. (1994) *Multiculturalism: Examining the Politics of Recognition*. Princeton, NJ: Princeton University Press.

Tsianakas, V. and Liamputtong, P. (2002) Prenatal testing: the perceptions and experiences of Muslim women in Australia, *Journal of Reproductive and Infant Psychology*, 20(1): 7–24.

2.3 Gender and socio-economic inequalities in mortality and health behaviours: an overview

Kate Hunt and G. David Batty

Introduction

Although some gender theorists have argued that gender should never be studied in isolation from social class and ethnicity, in reality empirical research on gender inequalities in health and socio-economic inequalities in health are rarely considered together. A review in the late 1990s noted that, in most of the inequalities literature, data for men and women were combined with adjustment for gender, included only one sex (usually men), or presented data for men and women separately with little comment on similarities or differences in the patterns of association (Macintyre and Hunt, 1997).

This chapter revisits the issue of gender and social inequalities in health. Its focus is on the UK, although international literature is drawn on where relevant. It first poses the question of why gender should still be important for health, and illustrates continuing gender disparities with UK data. It then discusses the complexities in researching interactions between gender and socio-economic inequalities in health before moving on to examine what recent evidence there is on gender and socio-economic inequalities in total and coronary heart disease mortality internationally. Finally, the chapter turns to two major risk factors for ill health (smoking and drinking) which are patterned by socio-economic position and contribute to gender differences in health. The way in which these behaviours are linked to 'presentations' of gender is demonstrated before recent evidence on the patterning of these behaviours by socio-economic position and gender in the UK is shown. Across the chapter as a whole, the aim is to demonstrate the complexities of the links between gender, social class and health.

Women's socio-economic position in relation to men

Why should gender still be important for health in the 21st century? Here we take the UK as an example of a high-income country; in general, gender inequalities are much more pronounced in low-income and middle-income countries. Gender equality legislation in the UK, such as the 1970 Equal Pay Act and the 1975 Sex Discrimination Act, extends back over more than three decades, culminating in the introduction of the Gender Equity Duty in 2007. Despite this, men's and women's lives still differ, exposing them to different social exposures, both materially and culturally. There are continuing gender inequalities in economic activity and labour market participation, education, earnings and other income, public participation and representation, and violent crime (Dench et al., 2002). For the purposes of understanding social class differences in health, gender differentials in engagement with paid work are perhaps of most direct relevance. Over the last 40 years, there has been a narrowing of the gap in economic activity between working-age men and women; by 2001, economic activity rates were 71 per cent for women and 84 per cent for men (Annandale and Hunt, 2000). However, horizontal and vertical segregation of the labour market remains in the UK, as in most countries. For example, in 2007, employed men were more likely to be working in skilled trades (19% men vs 2% women) and employed women in personal service (2% men vs 14% women). Gender differences also remain in part-time work, despite big reductions in the time women take out of the labour market to have and look after children. In 2007, 11 per cent of male and 42 per cent of female employees worked 30 hours or less a week (Self and Zealey, 2008).

Women continue to be paid less than men, in manual and non-manual occupations, whether or not they have dependent children, and in different educational strata (Self and Zealey, 2008). The gender pay gap, time spent in the workforce, and access to other sources of income all contribute to a lifetime income gap (that is, 'the price an average woman pays over the course of her working life for being female'; Dench et al., 2002) which has been estimated to be £250,000, plus another £140,000 if a woman has children.

As both occupation and material wealth are common bases for examining socio-economic inequalities, these differences in labour market engagement and reward suggest that we might expect to see different patterns of socio-economic inequalities in health for men and women. The workplace is also an important site for producing, reproducing and reinforcing both class and gender differentials (see, for example, Game and Pringle, 1983; Acker, 2006).

Social disadvantages of being female may lead to an expectation that women's health would be poorer than men's. However, the World Health Organization (WHO) has suggested that women's 'innate constitution' gives them an advantage over men, at least in relation to life expectancy (WHO, 1998). In the UK in 2005–7, life expectancy at birth was 81.5 for girls and 77.2 for boys, although the gender gap has narrowed in recent years (ONS, 2008). Although the causes of these well-documented differentials in male and female longevity are complex, international and historical patterns of gender differences in life expectancy suggest that the social world must interact with underlying biological differences (Doyal et al., 2001). Internationally, some of this variation is attributable to differences in the availability and quality of reproductive health care (Doyal, 2000). However, in countries where the health penalties of reproduction are much lower, some of the explanation for these changes over time lies in differences in behavioural risk factors (Charlton, 1997; Waldron, 2000) which are themselves linked to gender in intriguing ways, as we demonstrate later. Thus, the 'risky' nature of cultural constructions of masculinity are often suggested as the explanation for men's mortality disadvantage (Courtenay, 2000).

Complexities in researching the interactions between gender and socio-economic position in relation to health

Figure 2.3.1 provides a summary of the ways in which gender and health are linked. First, most cultures dichotomize gender and maximize differences between the genders (Figure 2.3.1, left-hand column). It is (often implicitly) assumed that men and women, male and female, masculine and feminine, will represent important axes of difference; Connell (1995: 4) refers to this as the 'commonsense knowledge [that] men and women act differently'. Second, there are different theoretical conceptualizations of gender: as fixed and static or as fluid and malleable, as structure or as role, as performance or achievement; as power, as distinct and distinguishable from sex (biology) or as inextricably interlinked. Whether we see these different conceptualizations of gender as competing or complementary, there is no doubt that

> there is now a more complex understanding of gender as a social reality... [each concept] of gender – as role, as performance, as institution – tries to include the dynamic and active construction

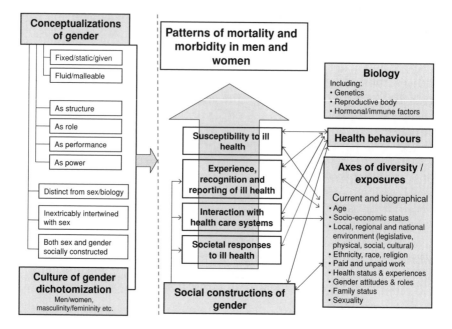

Figure 2.3.1 Sex/gender and health: conceptual underpinnings.
Source: adapted from Hunt (2007).

of gender ... at the same time, each tries to understand the persistence of gender as a social form (and thus, the focus on structure).
(Andersen, 2005: 441)

Irrespective of these different conceptual understandings of gender, our
ascribed sex and how this is interpreted in the culture within which we live
(gender) have consequences for our life chances, and hence our health. It is
a social fact that is repeatedly and universally noted throughout our lives.
Exactly *how* this process of classification and construction of social gender happens (and how this impacts on life chances and health) depends
on context: gender role expectations, family circumstances, occupational
opportunities and exposures, organizational structures, legislative pow-
ers, and broader historical, cultural and religious factors may all play their
part. Many of these factors are structured by socio-economic position.

If we consider the influence of gender on health (Figure 2.3.1, middle
column), gender differences may arise from differential susceptibility to ill
health; differential experience, recognition or reporting of ill health; differential family or societal responses to ill health; or differential responses
by, or uses of, the health care system for men and women (Hunt, 2007).
These factors in turn are influenced by an array of factors (Figure 2.3.1,

right-hand column), including biological mechanisms, differential adoption of health-related behaviours, and the interaction with exposures to other axes of diversity or inequality over the life course, with ethnicity and class often being identified as key axes of diversity in relation to gender (see, for example, Acker, 2006).

This complexity poses many challenges for researching the links between gender and health. Different methodologies lend themselves more naturally to different conceptualizations of gender. For example, while axes of diversity and inequality can be operationalized by current status and measures of lifetime exposure, as for example in research on exposure to adverse circumstances during childhood and adult life (Kuh et al., 2002), it is not easily possible to represent gender as a fluid, or situationally dependent, phenomenon in quantitative research. That gender concurrently has a 'peculiar omnipresence' and taken-for-grantedness or 'invisibility in most arenas of social life' (Lewis, 2007: 274) raises challenges for research on gender within all methodological paradigms.

Measuring socio-economic position in men and women

There has been debate about the best approach to measuring people's socio-economic position in society, both within health inequalities research and more broadly (see Hilary Graham's introductory chapter). In the last quarter of the 20th century, the measurement of social position among women was a particularly controversial issue. Measures based on education, housing tenure, occupation, income, absolute or relative material wealth, and area-based measures of deprivation have all been used; UK studies often use occupationally based measures; in Europe and the USA education is more commonly used. This range of measures complicates comparisons of social inequalities in men and women as there is evidence that the measure used differentially affects the strength of health gradients in men and women (Macintyre et al., 2003). For example, a study using both a measure of general socio-economic advantage and lifestyle and an occupationally based index showed that the extent of health inequality in women compared to men depended on the choice of measure (Sacker et al., 2000).

For many years, the Registrar General's classification system based on occupation was the most widely used measure of socio-economic position in the UK. However, it was subject to many criticisms, including its lack of a proper theoretical base, its failure to account for changes in the structure of occupations and its inability to adequately discriminate between women's occupations. Often the occupation of the 'head of household' was used. This meant that men were more often classified by their own occupation while married women were classified by their husband's occupation. There continues to be debate about whether individually-based or household-based measures are most appropriate in health research (e.g. Vagero, 2000).

Recent international evidence on socio-economic inequalities in mortality by gender

Prior to the last decade or so, the more limited inclusion of women in population-based studies meant that earlier systematic reviews of socio-economic position and health were often not generalizable to women (e.g. Gonzalez et al., 1998), although some studies which reported socio-economic gradients by gender noted different gradients in men and women (Kaplan and Keil, 1993). An earlier review of studies on socio-economic position, gender and health concluded that:

> in general, using conventional measures of socio-economic status... gradients in women's rates of death or health appear to be less steep and consistent than the gradients for men [although there are some] exceptions to the general pattern... [T]here is some evidence that CHD (coronary heart disease) mortality and morbidity may exhibit steeper gradients for women than for men... Emphasizing the pervasiveness of socio-economic and gender differences may, in general, have diverted attention from... whether gender differences in health are influenced by SES, and whether socio-economic gradients are influenced by gender.
>
> (Macintyre and Hunt, 1997: 326)

This review considered a range of health outcomes across studies, and did not take account of the impact of adjusting for risk factors for common diseases (for example, smoking, binge drinking and obesity). To examine international evidence on socio-economic inequalities in mortality by gender over the last decade, we undertook a systematic search for papers published since 1994. Given the suggestion that socio-economic gradients are steeper for men for all-cause mortality, but steeper for women for CHD mortality (Macintyre and Hunt, 1997), we sought to identify papers with data on both CHD and all-cause mortality. We used a three-pronged approach: a search of our own files; an electronic database search (described later); and scrutinization of the reference section of retrieved papers. The search was conducted in Medline via the Pubmed interface (http://www.ncbi.nlm.nih.gov/sites/entrez?db=PubMed), using 'socio-economic factors' and 'mortality' as Medical Subject Headings (MeSH) with 'cardiovascular diseases' or CHD, CVD (cardiovascular disease), IHD (ischemic heart disease) or heart disease in the title or abstract. This identified 560 papers. Titles, abstracts and, in some cases, full papers were examined to identify those which fulfilled the following criteria: (a) included all-cause and CHD mortality data by socio-economic status by gender, presented before and after adjustment for risk factors; (b) published in English from 1995 onwards; (c) the study was based on a prospective cohort design.

Only four studies (five publications) fulfilled these inclusion criteria (Pekkanen et al., 1995; Davey Smith et al., 1998; Hardarson et al., 2001; Steenland et al., 2002). All four were conducted in northern Europe (Finland, Iceland, Scotland) or the USA. Total and CHD mortality by socio-economic position and gender are presented in Table 2.3.1.[1] Two studies (Hardarson et al., 2001; Steenland et al., 2002) used education as the indicator of socio-economic position, and two used individual-level occupational social class (Pekkanen et al., 1995; Davey Smith et al., 1998). The most advantaged social group is the referent group in all but one study (Hardarson et al., 2001). The table allows comparison of gradients for all-cause and coronary mortality in men and women, before and after adjustment for preventable risk factors.

In three of the studies, there is some indication that gradients in all-cause mortality are stronger in men than in women in models adjusted only for age (Pekkanen et al., 1995; Davey Smith et al., 1998; Steenland et al., 2002); some of this weaker gradient in women may be accounted for by a reverse-class gradient in the incidence of breast cancer, although survival is greatest among the more affluent. In Finland's North Karelia Project, the hazard ratio (HR) for men classified as unskilled blue-collar workers in comparison with white-collar workers was 1.86 (equivalent HR for women 1.49); in the Scottish Renfrew and Paisley Study, the HR for men classified as unskilled blue-collar workers in comparison with white-collar workers was 1.52 (equivalent HR for women 1.32); and in the US Cancer Prevention Study, the HR for men with less than 9th-grade education in comparison with those with post-graduate education was 1.57 (equivalent HR for women 1.33). However, the confidence intervals for men and women overlapped in all but the Cancer Prevention Study. After adjustment for risk factors, there was only evidence for stronger socio-economic gradients in all-cause mortality for men in the Renfrew and Paisley Study and the Cancer Prevention Study.

For coronary mortality, trend statistics confirmed a stronger gradient for women than men in the Renfrew and Paisley study, both before adjustment for risk factors (HR women 1.50, p trend $= 0.0001$, HR men 1.33, p trend $= 0.002$) and after adjustment for risk factors (HR women 1.25, p trend $= 0.005$, HR men 1.16, p trend $= 0.13$). Somewhat stronger

Table 2.3.1 Prospective observational studies of men and women relating individual-level markers of socio-economic position (SEP) with all-cause and CHD mortality, with and without adjustment for risk factors

Study	Study description	Measure(s) of socio-economic position	Mortality outcome
North Karelia Project, Finland (Pekkanen et al., 1995)	Two Finnish population-based representative cohorts (comprising 8967 men, 9694 women) examined in 1972 or 1977 when aged 30–64 years; followed up for a maximum of 15 years	Individual-level occupational social class obtained through record linkage with census data: 1 = white collar 2 = skilled blue collar 3 = unskilled blue collar 4 = farmers	Record linkage with the National Death Registry for (1429 all cause deaths in men, 620 in women; 603 CHD deaths in men, 164 in women)
Renfrew and Paisley Study (Davey Smith et al., 1998)	Scottish population-based cohort (6961 men, 7991 women) examined between 1972 and 1976 when aged 45–64 years; followed up for 15 years	Individual-level Registrar General categorization of occupational social class based on self-report:[c] 1 = I/II 2 = III non-manual 3 = III manual 4 = IV and V	Record linkage with the National Death Registry (2133 all cause deaths in men, 1492 in women; CVD deaths 1143 in men, 726 in women)
Reykjavik Study (Hardarson et al., 2001)	Five Icelandic population-based cohort (9139 men, 9773 women) examined in 1967/9, 1970/2, 1974/9, 1979/84, and 1983/91 when aged 33–81 years; followed up for 4–30 years.	Self-report of individual-level educational attainment: 1 = elementary school or lower 2 = high school 3 = junior college 4 = university	Record linkage with the National Death Registry for (3175 all cause deaths in men, 2029 in women; 1257 CHD deaths in men, 469 in women)

| SEP–mortality* association (effect estimateˆ [95% CI]) | | | |
| Basic adjustment | | Adjustment for risk factor(s) | |
Men	Women	Men	Women
All cause	**All cause**	**All cause**	**All cause**
1 = referent [a]	1 = referent[a]	1 = referent[b]	1 = referent[b]
2 = 1.44 (1.22 1.70)	2 = 1.36 (1.06, 1.76)	2 = 1.29 (1.09 1.52)	2 = 1.14 (0.67, 1.96)
3 = 1.86 (1.55, 2.22)	3 = 1.49 (1.15, 1.92)	3 = 1.47 (1.23, 1.77)	3 = 1.66 (0.99, 2.79)
4 = 1.15 (0.97, 1.36)	4 = 1.23 (0.98, 1.54)	4 = 1.04 (0.88, 1.24)	4 = 1.24 (0.76, 2.03)
CHD	**CHD**	**CHD**	**CHD**
1 = referent[a]	1 = referent[a]	1 = referent[b]	1 = referent[b]
2 = 1.36 (1.06 1.74)	2 = 1.26 (0.74, 2.15)	2 = 1.18 (0.92, 1.52)	2 = 1.27 (0.98, 1.64)
3 = 1.54 (1.16, 2.02)	3 = 1.74 (1.05, 2.90)	3 = 1.22 (0.92, 1.61)	3 = 1.39 (1.07, 1.81)
4 = 1.10 (0.86, 1.41)	4 = 1.29 (0.81, 2.05)	4 = 0.99 (0.76, 1.287)	4 = 1.14 (0.89, 1.45)
All cause	**All cause**	**All cause**	**All cause**
1 = referent[a]	1 = referent[a]	1 = referent[c]	1 = referent[c]
2 = 1.25 (1.06, 1.47)	2 = 0.92 (0.77, 1.10)	2 = 1.13 (0.96, 1.34)	2 = 0.93 (0.78, 1.11)
3 = 1.40 (1.23, 1.60)	3 = 1.38 (1.17, 1.64)	3 = 1.18 (1.03, 1.34)	3 = 1.21 (1.02, 1.44)
4 = 1.52 (1.33, 1.74)	4 = 1.32 (1.14, 1.54)	4 = 1.22 (1.06, 1.40)	4 = 1.13 (0.97, 1.33)
p trend = 0.0001	*p* trend = 0.0001	*p* trend = 0.005	*p* trend = 0.014
CVD	**CVD**	**CVD**	**CVD**
1 = referent[a]	1 = referent[a]	1 = referent[c]	1 = referent[c]
2 = 1.23 (0.99, 1.54)	2 = 0.88 (0.68, 1.15)	2 = 1.13 (0.90, 1.41)	2 = 0.90 (0.69, 1.17)
3 = 1.35 (1.13, 1.60)	3 = 1.44 (1.12, 1.84)	3 = 1.20 (1.01, 1.44)	3 = 1.19 (0.93, 1.53)
4 = 1.33 (1.11, 1.60)	4 = 1.50 (1.20, 1.87)	4 = 1.16 (0.96, 1.39)	4 = 1.25 (0.99, 1.56)
p trend = 0.002	*p* trend = 0.0001	*p* trend = 0.13	*p* trend = 0.005
All cause	**All cause**	**All cause**	**All cause**
1 = referent[d]	1 = referent[d]	1 = referent[e]	1 = referent[e]
2 = 0.86 (0.79, 0.93)	2 = 0.79 (0.71, 0.87)	2 = 0.86 (0.80, 0.93)	2 = 0.86 (0.78, 0.95)
3 = 0.80 (0.71, 0.90)	3 = 0.65 (0.52, 0.81)	3 = 0.80 (0.71, 0.90)	3 = 0.71 (0.57, 0.89)
4 = 0.75 (0.65, 0.87)	4 = 0.74 (0.47, 1.15)	4 = 0.77 (0.66, 0.88)	4 = 1.29 (0.56, 1.35)
CAD	**CAD**	**CAD**	**CAD**
1 = referent[d]	1 = referent[d]	1 = referent[e]	1 = referent[e]
2 = 0.86 (0.76, 0.98)	2 = 0.66 (0.52, 0.82)	2 = 0.86 (0.76, 0.98)	2 = 0.79 (0.63, 0.98)
3 = 0.83 (0.69, 0.99)	3 = 0.45 (0.26, 0.78)	3 = 0.86 (0.71, 1.03)	3 = 0.56 (0.32, 0.97)
4 = 0.62 (0.48, 0.79)	4 = 0.84 (0.35, 2.02)	4 = 0.65 (0.50, 0.82)	4 = 1.29 (0.53, 3.12)

(continued)

Table 2.3.1 *(Continued)*

Study	Study description	Measure(s) of socio-economic position	Mortality outcome
Cancer Prevention Study (CPS II) (Steenland et al., 2002)	CPS II (499,265 men, 663,051 women) is a US population-based cohort examined in 1982 when aged 45–111 years; followed up for up to 14 years	Self-report of individual-level educational attainment: 1 = grammar school (<9th grade) 2 = some high school 3 = high school graduate 4 = some college 5 = college graduate 6 = post-graduate	Report by proxy, Cancer Society volunteer, or vital status data for CHD. In CPS II, there were 126,398 deaths in men, 104,421 in women

*CHD = coronary heart disease; CVD = coronary vascular disease; CAD = coronary artery disease; ^ hazard ratios
p trend = probability value for linear trend across socio-economic groups.
[a] adjusted for age.
[b] adjusted for age, smoking, cholesterol, hypertension, body mass index (BMI), physical activity.
[c] adjusted for DBP, cholesterol, BMI, FEV1, smoking, angina, ECG ischaemia and bronchitis.
[d] adjusted for age and calendar year.
[e] adjusted for age, calendar year, height, weight, total cholesterol, triglycerides, SBP, blood glucose and smoking.
[f] adjusted for age. Results presented are for the CPS-II; results are also available for CPS-I (1959–72) in which similar associations were seen, although gradients were weaker.
[g] adjusted for age, smoking, BMI, diet, alcohol, prevalent hypertension, and menopausal status (women). Results presented are for the CPS-II; results are also available for CPS-I (1959–72) in which similar associations were seen although gradients were weaker.

gradients in coronary mortality were also apparent for women than for men in the Cancer Prevention Study and the North Karelia Project, although confidence intervals for the estimates for men and women again overlapped. The Icelandic Reykjavik Study did not show any clear pattern for coronary mortality by socio-economic position.

It is surprising that so few studies published in the last decade fulfilled our relatively wide inclusion criteria, allowing a comparison by gender of the strength of gradients for all-cause and coronary mortality before and after adjustment for risk factors. It is hoped that the guidelines issued by the US National Institutes of Health (NIH) will initiate a culture change in the analysis and reporting of large-scale cohort studies by gender. In 1990 their guidelines mandated the inclusion of women and people from

SEP–mortality* association (effect estimate^ [95% CI])			
Basic adjustment		*Adjustment for risk factor(s)*	
Men	*Women*	*Men*	*Women*
All cause	**All cause**	**All cause**	**All cause**
1 = 1.57 (1.54, 1.61)	1 = 1.33 (1.29, 1.37)	1 = 1.28 (1.25, 1.31)	1 = 1.18 (1.15, 1.22)
2 = 1.59 (1.55, 1.62)	2 = 1.31 (1.28, 1.35)	2 = 1.30 (1.28, 1.33)	2 = 1.16 (1.13, 1.20)
3 = 1.37 (1.34, 1.39)	3 = 1.17 (1.14, 1.19)	3 = 1.20 (1.17, 1.22)	3 = 1.09 (1.07, 1.12)
4 = 1.30 (1.28, 1.33)	4 = 1.09 (1.06, 1.12)	4 = 1.16 (1.14, 1.19)	4 = 1.04 (1.01, 1.07)
5 = 1.09 (1.07, 1.12)	5 = 1.02 (0.99, 1.05)	5 = 1.04 (1.02, 1.06)	5 = 1.01 (0.98, 1.04)
6 = referent[f]	6 = referent[f]	6 = referent[g]	6 = referent[g]
CHD	**CHD**	**CHD**	**CHD**
1 = 1.62 (1.55, 1.69)	1 = 1.73 (1.62, 1.84)	1 = 1.31 (1.25, 1.36)	1 = 1.42 (1.33, 1.51)
2 = 1.68 (1.61, 1.75)	2 = 1.68 (1.58, 1.78)	2 = 1.37 (1.31, 1.43)	2 = 1.40 (1.32, 1.49)
3 = 1.46 (1.41, 1.51)	3 = 1.41 (1.33, 1.49)	3 = 1.27 (1.22, 1.32)	3 = 1.28 (1.20, 1.35)
4 = 1.35 (1.30, 1.40)	4 = 1.19 (1.12, 1.26)	4 = 1.20 (1.16, 1.25)	4 = 1.13 (1.06, 1.20)
5 = 1.10 (1.06, 1.15)	5 = 1.05 (0.98, 1.12)	5 = 1.06 (1.01, 1.10)	5 = 1.04 (0.97, 1.11)
6 = referent[f]	6 = referent[f]	6 = referent[g]	6 = referent[g]

ethnic minorities in all NIH-funded clinical research; from 1994 the guidelines also required analysis of clinical trial outcomes by sex. However, a review of research published in five leading American medical journals suggests that the shift towards routine analysis by gender was slow in the first decade after the guidelines were introduced (Vidaver et al., 2000). Given the changing patterns of risk factors in relation to both gender and class (some of which are explored later), it is important that the question of whether there are gender differences in socio-economic gradients in health (for cause-specific as well as all-cause mortality) continues to be revisited.

Smoking, gender and class

We now move from the patterning of mortality by gender and social class to consider how two major risk factors for premature mortality are intricately linked with gender and class. The first of these is smoking, a risk factor also discussed in Chapter 3.2.

Cigarette smoking typically establishes itself first among elite men, and thereafter works down class and status hierarchies (Greaves, 1996). Until the mid-1920s, smoking in Britain was largely a male habit (Elliot, 2008). Male consumption increased to the end of the Second World War, and fell substantially from the 1960s to the 1980s (Doll et al., 1997). Women only began to smoke on a large scale in Britain after cigarette advertisements directed at women began to appear in North America, the UK and other industrialized countries (Greaves, 1996). Female consumption increased rapidly from the Second World War until the 1970s when it began to fall, around ten years later than for men (Doll et al., 1997). National surveys from the early 1970s onwards demonstrate a diminution of gender differences alongside the dramatic reduction in the prevalence of smoking: in 1972, 52 per cent of men and 41 per cent of women smoked compared with 25 per cent of men and 23 per cent of women in 2005 (Goddard, 2006). Although gender differences in smoking in adults have reduced, more females than males smoke in adolescence (Amos and Bostock, 2007).

What is perhaps most remarkable about the link between gender and tobacco use is that smoking is linked to performances of gender identity in different cultures and countries. This includes countries at early stages of the 'smoking epidemic' when smoking is more clearly distinguished as a 'male' habit. For example, smoking is closely linked to the construction of masculinity among adolescent boys in Java, where 38 per cent of boys and 5 per cent of girls smoke (Ng et al., 2007), and in Scotland where equal numbers of men (29 per cent) and women (28 per cent) are smokers (Bramley et al., 2005).

Why is smoking so strongly linked to gender? Brandt (1996: 64), referring to the late 1920s, noted that the cigarette had 'remarkably elastic meanings' for both men and women and 'even managed to contain contradictory meanings'. The tobacco industry has exploited this plurality of connotations, making smoking a powerful way of 'doing gender' (West and Zimmerman, 1987). It has promoted smoking both as a symbol of masculinity (see Elliot, 2008) and of emancipation for women (Amos and Haglund, 2000). Greaves (1996: 20) argues that more sophisticated definitions of sexual equality from the 1930s allowed for 'six decades of elastic cultural definitions of women's smoking', and that the 'cultural meaning' of women's smoking altered 'from a symbol of being bought by men (prostitute), to being like men (lesbian/mannish/androgynous), to being able to attract men (glamorous/heterosexual)' (1996: 21–2).

Smoking also shows complex interrelationships with social class. Despite the downward trend in smoking in the UK, the prevalence of smoking in people from the most disadvantaged circumstances has fallen little in recent decades and, as yet, there is little evidence that tobacco control policies in the UK are undermining the link between social disadvantage and smoking (see Chapter 3.2). Smoking in Britain is increasingly 'a habit acquired and sustained by those who occupy disadvantaged positions within the social hierarchy' (Graham, 1994: 102) and is identified as 'an important component of differences in mortality between social classes' (Acheson, 1998: 83).

Qualitative work has demonstrated the highly complex ways in which class and gender interact in relation to smoking. Graham (1994: 121) has described how smoking is

> enmeshed in the strategies by which women experience and sur-
> vive inequality... [It] is a way of living with and living through
> the experiences that go with social inequality. In the context of
> gender and class oppression, it provides a resource which can be
> accessed instantly when caring responsibilities are many and ma-
> terial resources are few.

These subtle, but powerful, links are more easily demonstrated in qualitative than quantitative research given the complex and changing links
between tobacco consumption, gender and class over the 20th century
(Hunt et al., 2004). Nonetheless, it is important to continue to examine
the prevalence of smoking by social class and gender given the contribution of smoking to avoidable mortality.

Alcohol, gender and class

Alcohol-related deaths in the UK increased from 4144 in 1991 to 8758
in 2006, despite a stable population base. Throughout this period, male
rates were substantially higher and the gender gap increased, culminating
in a male death rate of 18.3 per 100,000 and 8.8 per 100,000 for females
in 2006 (Self and Zealey, 2008). Alcohol-related deaths were highest in
the most deprived areas, and this relationship was stronger for men than
women. For men, the alcohol-related death rate in the 5 per cent most
deprived areas was 31.9 deaths per 100,000 compared with 6.2 deaths
per 100,000 in the 5 per cent least deprived areas; equivalent figures for
women were 11.3 per 100,000 and 3.7 per 100,000 (Self and Zealey, 2008).
However, the relationship between alcohol and socio-economic position
varies depending on the measure of consumption used. For example, men
and women from households with higher gross weekly incomes were more
likely to drink in the previous week than others, but there is little variation
in the proportion who consumed more than recommended daily levels
on at least one day in the week prior to interview (Self and Zealey, 2008).
Drinking has been described as 'without doubt, a gendered behaviour'
(McPherson et al., 2004: 738). Higher levels of alcohol consumption are related to negative 'masculine' characteristics (such as aggression) and lower
levels of consumption are related to positive 'masculine' characteristics
(such as instrumentality) and positive 'feminine' characteristics (such as
nurturance) among both women and men (see, for example, Ricciardelli
et al., 2001). However, the links between 'masculinity', 'femininity' and
alcohol consumption are complex.

In high-income Western nations, binge drinking is more common among younger people, particularly younger men (Kuntsche et al., 2004). There is debate about whether levels of binge drinking in young men and women are converging (e.g. McPherson et al., 2004; Emslie et al., 2009). It has been argued that 'the cultural interpretation of alcohol as masculine has proliferated for centuries' (Lemle and Mishkind, 1989: 215). This is particularly true for heavy drinking, and qualitative research shows that being able to drink excessively and hold one's drink are important elements of traditional masculinity (de Visser and Smith, 2007), although excessive drinking among (young) women has become more visible as it has received more attention in the popular media (Day et al., 2004; Lyons et al., 2006). Nonetheless, marked gender differences in alcohol consumption remain, both at younger and older ages (Plant et al., 2002; Emslie et al., 2009).

As women's drinking becomes more common, we might expect that heavy drinking becomes less associated with cultural constructions of masculinity. However, as with smoking, it appears that increasingly complex ways of promoting distinctions in the ways that heavy drinking is associated with gender are developing. For example, a review of coverage of alcohol in magazines targeted at men concluded that 'great effort appeared to be going into men's magazines to construct men's drinking in different ways to women's drinking' (Lyons et al., 2006: 230).

Current quantitative evidence from the UK on socio-economic patterning of smoking and drinking by gender

Evidence on social inequalities in smoking by gender is shown in Figures 2.3.2 and 2.3.3, drawn from a survey designed to provide a representative sample of the population living in private households in England (Sproston and Primatesta, 2004). The measures of socio-economic position presented here are equivalized household income and the UK's new National Statistics Socio-economic Classification (NS SEC) (see Hilary Graham's introductory chapter).

In 2003, 27 per cent of men and 23 per cent of women were current smokers, although the prevalence was much higher in young adults than at older ages (less than 10% of men and women aged 75 and over were smokers). Clear socio-economic gradients for smoking are evident for both men and women (Figures 2.3.2 and 2.3.3). For both genders, these were more pronounced using equivalized household income to measure socio-economic position (Figure 2.3.3) than occupational social class of the household reference person (Figure 2.3.2), but the magnitude of the gradients was similar in men and women. (For household-equivalized income,

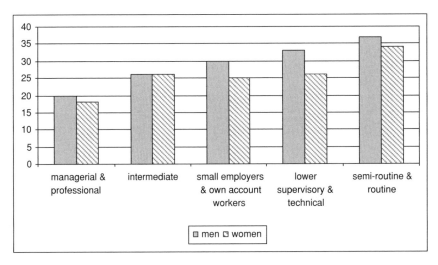

Figure 2.3.2 Proportion (%) of current smokers by socio-economic position (NS-SEC) of household reference person and sex, England, 2003.
Source: Sproston and Primatesta (2004), Table 3.3.

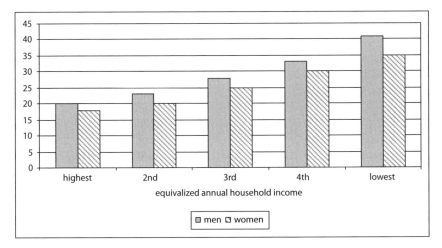

Figure 2.3.3 Proportion (%) of current smokers by income quintile (based on equivalized annual household income) and sex, England, 2003.
Source: Sproston and Primatesta (2004), Table 3.4.

there was a 14-percentage point difference between the highest and lowest quintiles for men, and a 13-point difference for women; for occupational social class, there was a 15-point difference between men from managerial and professional households and a 14-point difference for women).

Binge drinking has been shown to increase the risk of coronary heart disease in both men and women (Kauhanen et al., 1997). It is therefore the measure of alcohol consumption that we examine here. Binge drinkers were defined as those who reported drinking at least twice the recommended daily limit (i.e. in excess of 8 units for men and 6 units for women). There was no clear graded relationship between binge drinking and either measure of socio-economic position in men or women (see Figures 2.3.4 and 2.3.5), although more women from the least advantaged households were classed as binge drinkers (28% where household reference person was in a semi-routine or routine job; 20% where equivalized household income was in the lowest quintile).

Conclusion

This chapter has discussed the importance of examining socio-economic gradients in health by gender in order to better understand their causes.

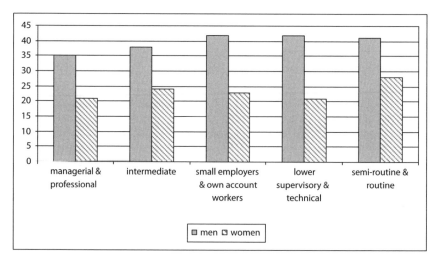

Figure 2.3.4 Proportion (%) of binge drinking on heaviest drinking day in past week by socio-economic position (NS-SEC) of household reference person and sex, England, 2003.
Source: Sproston and Primatesta (2004), Table 2.7.

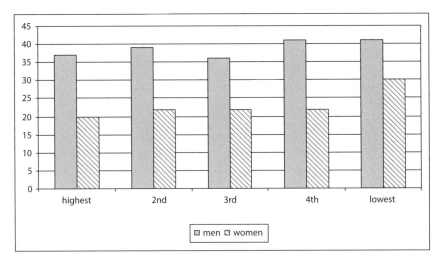

Figure 2.3.5 Proportion (%) of binge drinking on heaviest drinking day in past week by income quintile (based on equivalized annual household income) and sex, England, 2003.
Source: Sproston and Primatesta (2004), Table 2.8.

When total and CVD mortality are the outcomes of interest, there are disappointingly few well-designed and sufficiently powered studies examining this issue. This does not necessarily reflect an absence of data but rather how data are presented. That is, results are often pooled by gender. Further research is needed to carefully examine whether social gradients in health are changing in the same ways for men and women. This has added importance given the changing patterns of risk factors which will ultimately impact upon health in relation to gender and socio-economic position, and the subtlety of the ways in which important health behaviours continue to be a means of demonstrating gender competency or 'doing gender'. The challenge remains to bring together research on gender inequalities in health and socio-economic inequalities in health, but there is perhaps an even greater challenge in integrating insights on the links between gender, class and health (and health behaviours) from different methodological traditions.

Note

1. Results from a later paper by Steenland et al. (2004) are not included as analyses are of a sub-group of those included in their earlier paper.

Acknowledgements

Kate Hunt is funded by the Medical Research Council (MRC) Social and Public Health Sciences Unit (WBS no. U1300.00.004). G. David Batty is a Wellcome Trust Fellow. Thanks to Vittoria Lutje for conducting the literature search.

References

Acheson, D. (1998) *Independent Inquiry into Inequalities in Health Report.* London: The Stationery Office.

Acker, J. (2006) Inequality regimes: gender, class, in organizations, *Gender and Society*, 20: 441–64.

Amos, A. and Bostock, Y. (2007) Young people, smoking and gender – a qualitative exploration, *Health Education Research*, 22(6): 770–81.

Amos, A. and Haglund, M. (2000) From social taboo to 'torch of freedom': the marketing of cigarettes to women, *Tobacco Control*, 9: 3–8.

Andersen, M.L. (2005) Thinking about women. A quarter century's view, *Gender and Society*, 19(4): 437–55.

Annandale, E., and Hunt, K. (2000) Gender inequalities in health: research at the cross-roads, in E. Annandale and K. Hunt (eds) *Gender Inequalities in Health*. Buckingham: Open University Press.

Bramley, C., Sproston, K. and Shelton, N. (2005) *The Scottish Health Survey 2003: Volume 2, Adults*. Edinburgh: Scottish Executive.

Brandt, A.M. (1996) Recruiting women smokers: the engineering of consent, *JAMWA*, 51, 63–6.

Charlton, J. (1997) *The Health of Adult Britain: 1841–1994. Office for National Statitistics Decennial Supplement*. London: HMSO.

Connell, R. (1995) *Masculinities*. Cambridge: Polity Press.

Courtenay, W. (2000). Constructions of masculinity and their influence on men's well-being: a theory of gender and health, *Social Science and Medicine*, 50: 1385–401.

Darey Smith, G., Hart, C., Watt, G. et al. (1998) Individual social class, area-based deprivation, cardiovascular disease risk factors, and mortality: the Renfrew and Paisley Study, *Journal of Epidemiology and Community Health*, 52: 399–405.

Day, K., Gough, B., and McFadden, M. (2004) 'Warning! Alcohol can seriously damage your feminine health': a discourse analysis of recent British newspaper coverage of women and drinking, *Feminist Media Studies*, 4: 165–82.

de Visser, R., and Smith, J.A. (2007) Alcohol consumption and masculine identity among young men, *Psychology and Health*, 22(5): 595–614.

Dench, S., Aston, J., Evans, C. et al. (2002) *Key Indicators of Women's Position in Britain*. London: Department of Trade and Industry.

Doll, R., Derby, S., and Whitley, E. (1997) Trends in mortality from smoking-related diseases, in J. Charlton (ed.) *The Health of Adult Britain: 1841–1994*. London: Office for National Statistics.

Doyal, L. (2000) Gender equity in health: debates and dilemmas, *Social Science and Medicine*, 51: 931–9.

Doyal, L., Hunt, K. and Payne, S. (2001) Sex, gender and non-communicable diseases: an overview of issues and recent evidence. Report prepared for the NCD cluster of the World Health Organization.

Elliot, R. (2008) *Women and Smoking since 1890*. Abingdon: Routledge.

Emslie, C., Lewars, H., Batty, G.D. and Hunt, K. (2009) Are there gender differences in levels of heavy, binge and problem drinking? Evidence from three generations in the west of Scotland, *Public Health*, 123: 12–14.

Game, A. and Pringle, R. (1983) *Gender at Work*. Sydney: George Allen and Unwin.

Goddard, E. (2006) *General Household Survey 2006: Smoking and Drinking in Adults, 2005*. London: Office for National Statistics.

Gonzalez, M.A., Artalejo, F.R. and Calero, J.d.R. (1998) Relationship between socioeconomic status and ischaemic heart disease in cohort and case-control studies: 1960–1993, *International Journal of Epidemiology*, 27: 350–8.

Graham, H. (1994) Surviving by smoking, in S. Wilkinson, and C. Kitzinger (eds) *Women and Health: Feminist Perspectives*. London: Taylor & Francis.

Greaves, L. (1996) *Smoke Screen: Women's Smoking and Social Control*. London: Scarlet Press.

Hardarson, T., Gardarsdottir, M., Gudmundsson, K.T. et al. (2001) The relationship between educational level and mortality: the Reykjavik study, *Journal of Internal Medicine*, 249: 495–502.

Hunt, K. (2007) Understanding gender and health: systematically comparing the health and health experiences of men and women [PhD]. *MRC Social and Public Health Sciences Unit*. Glasgow: University of Glasgow.

Hunt, K., Hannah, M.K. and West, P. (2004) Contextualising smoking: masculinity, femininity and class differences in smoking in men and women from three generation in the west of Scotland, *Health Education Research Theory and Practice*, 19: 239–49.

Kaplan, G.A. and Keil, J. (1993) Socioeconomic factors and cardiovascular disease: a review of the literature, *Circulation*, 88: 1973–98.

Kauhanen, J., Kaplan, G.A., Goldberg, D. and Salonen, J.T. (1997) Beer binging and mortality: results from the Kuopio ischaemic heart disease risk factor study, a prospective population based study, *British Medical Journal*, 315: 846–51.

Kuh, D., Hardy, R., Langenberg, C., Richards, M. and Wadsworth, M. (2002) Mortality in adults aged 26–54 years related to socio-economic conditions in childhood and adulthood: post war birth cohort study, *British Medical Journal*, 325: 1076–80.

Kuntsche, E., Rehm, N. and Gmel, G. (2004) Characteristics of binge drinkers in Europe, *Social Science* and *Medicine*, 59: 113–27.

Lemle, R. and Mishkind, M.E. (1989) Alcohol and masculinity, *Journal of Substance Abuse Treatment*, 6: 213–22.

Lewis, L. (2007) Epistemic authority and the gender lens, *Sociological Review*, 55(2): 273–92.

Lyons, A., Dalton, S.I. and Hoy, A. (2006) 'Hardcore drinking': portrayals of alcohol consumption in young women's and men's magazines, *Journal of Health Psychology*, 11: 223–32.

Macintyre, S. and Hunt, K. (1997) Socioeconomic position, gender and health; how do they interact? *Journal of Health Psychology*, 2: 315–34.

Macintyre, S., McKay, L., Der, G. and Hiscock, R. (2003) Socio-economic position and health: what you observe depends on how you measure it, *Journal of Public Health Medicine*, 25(4): 288–94.

McPherson, M., Casswell, S. and Pledger, M. (2004) Gender convergence in alcohol consumption and related problems: issues and outcomes from comparisons of New Zealand survey data, *Addiction*, 99(6): 738–48.

Ng, N., Weinehall, L. and Ohman, A. (2007) 'If I don't smoke, I'm not a real man': Indonesian teenage boys' views about smoking, *Health Education Research*, 22(6): 794–804.

Office for National Statistics (ONS) (2008) *Life Expectancy*. London: Office for National Statistics.

Pekkanen, J., Tuomilehto, J., Uutela, A., Vartiainen, E. and Nissinen, A. (1995) Social class, health behaviour, and mortality among men and women in eastern Finland, *British Medical Journal*, 311: 589–93.

Plant, M., Plant, M. and Mason, W. (2002) Drinking, smoking and illicit drug use among British adults: gender differences explored, *Journal of Substance Use*, 7: 24–33.

Ricciardelli, L.A., Connor, J.P., Williams, R.J. and Young, R.M. (2001) Gender stereotypes and drinking cognitions as indicators of moderate and high risk drinking among young women and men, *Drug and Alcohol Dependence*, 61: 129–36.

Sacker, A., Firth, D., Fitzpatrick et al. (2000) Comparing health inequality in men and women: prospective study of mortality 1986–96, *British Medical Journal*, 320: 1303–07.

Self, A. and Zealey, L. (2008) *Social Trends 38*. Basingstoke: Palgrave Macmillan.

Sproston, K. and Primatesta, P. (2004) *Health Survey for England 2003. Volume 1*. London: The Stationery Office.

Steenland, K., Henley, J. and Thun, M. (2002) All-cause mortality and cause-specific death rates by educational status for two million people in two American Cancer Society cohorts, 1959–1996, *American Journal of Epidemiology*, 156(1): 11–21.

Steenland, K., Henley, J., Calle, E. and Thun, M. (2004) Individual- and area-level socioeconomic status variables as predictors of mortality in a cohort of 179,393 persons, *American Journal of Epidemiology*, 159(11): 1047–56.

Vagero, D. (2000) Health inequalities in women and men: studies of specific causes of death should use household criteria, *British Medical Journal*, 320: 1286–87.

Vidaver, R.M., Lafleur, B., Tong, C. et al. (2000) Women subjects in NIH-funded clinical research literature: lack of progress in both representation and analysis by sex, *Journal of Women's Health and Gender-based Medicine*, 9(5): 495–504.

Waldron, I. (2000) Trends in gender differences in mortality: relationships to changing gender differences in behaviour and other causal factors, in E. Annandale and K. Hunt (eds) *Gender Inequalities in Health*. Buckingham: Open University Press.

West, C. and Zimmerman, D. (1987) Doing gender, *Gender and Society*, 1: 125–51.

World Health Organization (WHO) (1998). *Gender and Health: Technical Paper*. Geneva: WHO.

2.4 Class cultures and the meaning of young motherhood

Naomi Rudoe and Rachel Thomson

Introduction

The UK continues to have the highest teenage fertility rate in Western Europe, and the third highest rate, after the USA and New Zealand, in countries forming the Organization for Economic Co-operation and Development (UNICEF, 2007). Early childbearing is seen as problematic in industrialized societies because of the 'disparity between readiness for sexual activity and the socially approved timing of its expression and consequences' and because of the economic strain on society (Wellings et al., 1999: 184). Yet in historical terms, rates of early motherhood in the UK have remained relatively stable over the course of the twentieth century, the main change being that these births increasingly occur outside marriage (Joshi, 2008).

The overall pattern in fertility rates points to a gradual rise in the age at which women have their first child, with patterns in childbearing reflecting the diverging biographical patterns of women's lives (discussed in Hilary Graham's introductory chapter). Later childbearing is associated with participation in higher education and full-time careers, and earlier childbearing with socio-economic deprivation, lower levels of educational qualification, and low-paid and part-time work (Ferri and Smith, 2003; Joshi, 2008). In the context of these diverging pathways into motherhood, teenage motherhood is considered particularly problematic (McRobbie, 2004; Thomson et al., 2008). Contemporary representations often cast teenage mothers in negative terms (Tyler, 2008), as irresponsibly opting out of education and onto reliance on state benefits. Analyses of social exclusion tend to reinforce such views by documenting how early motherhood contributes to the transmission of disadvantage across the life course (childhood disadvantage leading to early motherhood and on to adult disadvantage) and across generations (from parent to child) (Hobcraft and Kiernan, 2001; Bynner et al., 2002).

Early motherhood continues to be normative in some communities: more common among Afro-Caribbean, Pakistani and Bangladeshi women than among white women, with evidence suggesting that most of Asian women are married when they give birth (Berthoud, 2001). Geographical variation is also significant in factors influencing teenage pregnancy: social deprivation has been found to explain about three-quarters of the area variation in teenage conceptions and abortions in England and Wales, with service provision likely to account for the remaining variation (Bradshaw et al., 2005). The percentage of teenage conceptions leading to abortion is inversely correlated with deprivation, so that with the exception of London, 'the proportion of conceptions leading to abortion in the least deprived wards is approximately twice that in the most deprived for each region' (Uren et al., 2007: 38). This variation in the abortion rate may be explained by accessibility to abortion services at a local level (Bradshaw et al., 2005), but young women's decision making is also influenced by young women's socio-economic circumstances, family and community views (Lee et al., 2004).

In this chapter, we draw on qualitative research to challenge dominant understandings of teenage motherhood. We argue that there is a 'logic of practice' that means that becoming a teenage parent continues to make sense for some young women, a logic that goes beyond sexual behaviour and decision making to include wider life chances and local cultures of value. How teenage parenthood is understood depends on the perspective from which it is encountered. Our argument draws particularly on our own research, including published studies (Thomson, 2000) and previously unpublished research with young mothers (Rudoe, in press). Using insights from these studies, we illustrate the 'logic of practice' within which teenage parenthood is given meaning, and then interrogate three assumptions about teenage pregnancy: that teenage parenthood always disrupts education, that the teenage years are the wrong time to become a mother, and that teenage pregnancy is always a mistake. We begin by briefly highlighting the links between social disadvantage and teenage motherhood before introducing the qualitative studies which inform the chapter.

Social inequality and young motherhood

The knowledge base for policy in the UK draws heavily on quantitative data that confirm the significance of socio-economic and educational status in relation to teenage sexual activity and childbearing. Data from the second *National Survey of Sexual Attitudes and Lifestyles* showed a significant association between educational level and motherhood at younger than 18 years: 29 per cent of sexually active young women in the study who left school at 16 without qualifications had a child by the time they were 17 (compared to 14% of those leaving school at 16 with qualifications and to 1% of those remaining in education after 16) (Wellings et al., 2001). The study also found that young people 'who leave school later, with qualifications, are less likely to have early intercourse, more likely to use contraception at first sex, be sexually competent,[1] and (for women) less likely to become pregnant if they have sex' (Wellings et al., 2001: 1850).

Policies equating teenage pregnancy with social exclusion have tended to rely on quantitative research evidence, neglecting qualitative research findings in the process (Graham and McDermott, 2005). It is important that early parenthood is placed within a broader context that captures how youth transitions have been changing differentially in response to wider social and economic changes, with the shift towards extended transitions more a feature of middle-class transitions and of some ethnic groups. Studies into youth transitions in Britain over recent decades have indicated that young people are economically dependent for longer on their parents and struggle to achieve adult identities (Jones, 2005; Furlong and Cartmel, 2007; Henderson et al., 2007). This 'extended dependency' represents inter-generational continuity for the middle class but is a new biographical pattern for working-class young people (or the socially mobile 'new' middle class). Factors shaping this change include the diminishing of the youth labour market over the past three decades, together with a reduction in state benefits and an emphasis on entering further or higher education (MacDonald and Marsh, 2005). A minority of young people continue to experience 'accelerated' transitions to adulthood. These tend to be young people with little family support and/or who are on the margins of the labour market. The 'fast lane' to adulthood is a route epitomized by the teenage mother (Bynner et al., 2002).

The 'logic' of early parenthood

Where quantitative approaches tend to describe and explain a social problem, qualitative approaches can interrogate how and why such behaviour makes sense to those involved. The concept of a 'logic of practice' is taken from the work of Pierre Bourdieu (1980), and points to the internal and local logics of cultural practices. Bourdieu's approach illustrates how resources (what he terms capital) may or may not be converted into symbolic value, or power, and thus how inequalities are reproduced. So for example, a certain kind of education is a resource that has value and may be converted into other kinds of value, such as career, and access to social circles. However, some kinds of resources do not travel so easily; they 'do not operate as forms of capital ... but do have value for those who use and make them' (Skeggs, 2004: 17). For example, 'toughness' may be a valuable resource for a young man living in an inner-city environment, yet it may not be something that can be converted into a resource with value beyond that location (for example, toughness may be negatively viewed within the education system and by potential employers). Similarly, youthful fertility can be seen as a resource, the value of which is tied to a particular social location.

In understanding these 'logics of practice', it is important to remember that not all teenage motherhood occurs in the context of socially deprived communities, and working-class young mothers do not uniformly value parenting over education or employment. Simon Duncan (2005) elaborates this point by arguing that, although social class is 'materially just as important as ever', and there are class-based differences in primarily mother/primarily worker identities, these are not simply divided between working and middle classes, but 'refer to more nuanced social identities' (2005: 73). Mothers' choices are structured 'through the development of career as an identity, through biographical experience, through relations with partners, and through the development of normative views in social networks. In this way they become social moralities . . . [which] are geographically and historically articulated' (2005: 73).

An illustration of the way in which attitudes towards early motherhood fit within wider logics of practice is provided by a study of young people's values undertaken by one of us (Rachel Thomson) and colleagues. This multi-method study combined questionnaires ($n = 1800$), focus groups ($n = 56$) and interviews ($n = 43$), capturing the broader moral landscape against which attitudes towards sexual activity and early parenthood take shape within five contrasting localities within the UK (Thomson, 2000). Here we highlight the meanings of early parenthood for students attending Forest Green, a comprehensive school in an affluent middle-class commuter town, and North Park, a comprehensive school within a disadvantaged public housing estate.

One of the prompts used in focus groups discussion in this study was the proposition that the age of consent for heterosexual sex should be lowered from the age of 16 to 14. The middle-class young people in Forest Green reacted to this proposal in a hostile way, insisting on the importance of maintaining a correct sequence to the events of the future. Teenage sex should not happen before young people are 'ready' for it:

Miles:[2] I think it's sort of like a bit stupid at the moment because like 16 is like – you can get on with 16 year olds on their sixteenth birthday – you know – and have sex and then the next nine months, before they're 17, they have a baby and then they haven't even finished school yet – they'd just be like in the lower sixth and then they've sort of got this baby on their hands and they haven't even like . . . not even have a first boyfriend or a husband like – they'd have to either quit school or put it up for adoption which is . . . sort of like immature.

(young man, aged 12–13, male group)

Girls agreed that there was 'nothing grown up about having sex', explaining that sex should be special and that pregnancy was too big a risk. Not only did young people believe that it was necessary to wait for the right moment for sex, but also that

Heather: If you really want to have a child then you should be able to wait till that child's ready to come and [giggles] sorry, appear. You should be in a stable relationship – at least at the beginning of a child's life.

(young woman, aged 15–16, mixed group)

Young people at Forest Green school admired educational success, individuality and sociability – qualities that can be understood as forms of cultural capital, acquired in the present and realized in the future. Such deferred dividends were challenged by competing notions of value that operated in the immediacy of here and now – the physical capital of attractiveness and sexual experience:

Susanna: And like if you're a teenager and you get pregnant it doesn't necessarily just because you couldn't support it – necessarily mean you shouldn't have it because once you're pregnant then it would be your decision, and it's not up to anyone else to make that for you.

Joe: If like a pikey had a baby or something then you can't . . .

INTERVIEWER (INT): A what?

Nick: A pikey.

Joe: A pikey had a baby or something then you can't just let the child grow up in that environment 'cos that's bad.

Richard: You'd have to take him AWAY.

INT: What kind of environment does a pikey live in?

Joe: Grows up with loads of drugs and things round him.

Lorna: It's got to be a nice environment though.

Nick: They steal everything, take drugs and things like that.

Richard: Burnt out cars in the driveway.

Lorna: Bricks through the window.

Nick: Yeah.

Lorna: And they gave up school five years ago.

Nick: About 10 years old when they left school.

Richard: They'll all be smoking in the house – they wouldn't actually care there's a baby – they'd all be like smoking and feeding it 'Happy Shopper' food.
Nick: Happy Shopper [laughter] My Nan uses Happy Shopper!
(aged 14–15, mixed group)

By demonizing those they describe as 'pikeys', pregnancy, parenthood and dependency are placed beyond the pale for these young people. They are not things they need to imagine or explore strategies to deal with. Having a child without also being able to support it is not included as a possible future.

The same proposal gave rise to a very different discussion in North Park, a school located within an economically disadvantaged public housing estate in the north of England. While the key tension for young people in Forest Green lay in the boundary between values that dominated the present and values which could only be realized in the future, tensions in North Park surrounded the interface between the female-dominated spaces of the home and the male-dominated spaces of the streets, pubs and parties. For young women in particular, sexuality and sexual attraction mark the interface between these private and public fields, holding and expressing the contradictions between competing values and sources of authority. Thus it was common to find young women who simultaneously experienced themselves as powerful and vulnerable in relation to male partners, depending on where their identities were located:

Kerry: I think they think a lot of everything is the girl's fault be-cause a lot of girls nowadays are the ones that make the first move or the ones that like start talking to the lads rather than the lads talking to the girls – 'cos there's a lot of boys that are now weaker – like physically – no, mentally weaker – like shy and . . .
Rose: Lads that are shy.
Kerry: Rather than the girls – they just, 'Oh, I'll talk to anyone, me'.
INT: Yea. So what happens to the shy lads then . . .
Kerry: I'll get you set up with her, I'll do this for you – yet it's the girls that's finally got to go and ask him really.
INT: So the girls have to make things happen then, do they?
Rose: Yea.
Kerry: A lot of the time but then other times there's like some not so shy ones and they'll just jump on you [laughter].
(aged 13–14, female group)

Older or more experienced men posed particular problems. These con-cerns were voiced in discussions of lowering the age of consent from 16 to 14:

INT: Do you think it's to do with age?

Amy: It's to do with experience 'cos – some people are more mature when they're younger than they are when they're older.

Teresa: It's to do with experience 'cos you might not know.

Louise: When you first have it, you haven't got experience [...]

Teresa: Because, like, you could go out somewhere or a party or somewhere and you could have, like, one too many and all that and a man might – of thirty or something like that – could just jump into bed with you just because you was fourteen and all that.

(aged 12–13, female group)

Mothers and grandmothers provided clear advice to their daughters to avoid the traps created by these contradictions, telling girls to 'watch out', 'you're too clever to be stupid' and 'you're going to have more fun than we did'. But though young people relayed this advice, they were not necessarily able to resolve the contradictions between private and public worlds any better than their mothers before them.

While the compromising of agency involved in heterosexual relations may be temporarily problematic, parenthood provides a certain path to the accumulation of experience – a concrete and local vision of the future that was consistent with their values. In Bourdieu's terms, there was an internal logic to the practice of early parenthood in that it was supported by their objective circumstances. This could be seen in the subsequent anchoring of the discussions of parenthood in time and space through the experience of friends and family, leaving the career and travel plans as abstract dreams (Nilsen, 1999):

Teresa: 'Cos my next door neighbour's daughter – she was only sixteen – and she had a baby but she's saying that, I would have liked to have gone out – but she said she wouldn't change any-thing for him now because she said she loves him and everything and – her little baby – she says she loves him but she wouldn't change it back but she would have liked to have gone out and had a bit more of a life.

Rachel: My sister still goes out even though she has two kids.

Adel: No, my sister can get people to babysit.

Ronnie: My sister's had her second last week.

(age 12–13, female group)

Parenthood lies at the centre of most young people's visions of their future, even if it is to be delayed by career and education (Henderson et al., 2007). Although young people in North Park expressed many of the same opinions as those in Forest Green about the problems posed by teenage parenthood, their discussions were based on a grounded knowledge of coping strategies and the absence of belief in a couple relationship underpinning parenthood. Motherhood meant juggling competing demands within a limited time frame:

> *INT:* Do you think it's difficult to have a career and to have kids and ...
> *Donna:* Yea, 'cos then you might not have time for the kids.
> *Sonia:* Yea, might just keep doing it and doing it till you're too old to have a kid.
> (aged 14–15, female group)

Attitudes towards abortion also play a part. They were generally disapproving in North Park, with only 42 per cent indicating that abortion was ever acceptable in contrast to the 75 per cent in Forest Green who expressed this view. Given the absence of strong religious affiliations in either site, it could be argued that these attitudes are an indication of the desirability of motherhood and an acceptance of a collective future involving mutual dependency. Where motherhood is valued more highly than paid work, where being single and sexually available is a disempowering condition and where the couple relationship is not to be relied on, it can make sense to change the sequence of the stages of autonomy, to disrupt the order – to have a baby before you've had the first boyfriend.

Challenging dominant perspectives on early parenthood

Empirical studies have investigated teenage pregnancy and motherhood in relation to social inclusion and exclusion, education, housing, support networks and the care system (see Walkerdine et al., 2001; Letherby et al., 2002; Mitchell and Green, 2002; Arai, 2003; Kidger, 2004; Wiggins et al., 2005; Dawson and Hosie, 2005; Hirst et al., 2006; Cater and Coleman, 2006; Alldred and David, 2007; Barn and Mantovani, 2007; Cooke and Owen, 2007). In the remainder of this chapter we examine how the findings from qualitative research with pregnant young women and young mothers can disrupt certain assumptions that are prevalent in relation to teenage motherhood, focusing on three in turn. The data presented come from doctoral research conducted by one of us (Naomi Rudoe) in 2007–8 at an alternative educational setting in London staffed by dedicated professionals, where 16–19-year-old pregnant young women study a modular course involving preparation for childbirth and motherhood, as well as life skills, literacy and numeracy (Rudoe, in press). The majority of the young women attending the setting were of Black Caribbean,

White and Black Caribbean, or Black African parentage. This study combines participant observation and interviews as a way of capturing the subjective experiences of young mothers. The excerpts presented are taken from individual semi-structured interviews with a focus on pregnancy and motherhood.

Teenage parenting as disruptive of educational pathways?

A major policy concern in relation to teenage pregnancy is the way it disrupts young women's education. While we are not downplaying the barriers to study that motherhood may create, young women do not always tell a story about their pregnancy as an interruption to their education. Many who become pregnant have been excluded from school or are self-excluded, and do not want to return to mainstream school (Hosie and Selman, 2006). Even those who are following a vocational course of study at college may not perceive their pregnancy as a disruption to their educational plans. Taylor, a 17-year-old pregnant young woman of Ghanaian and Caribbean parentage, had had an abortion at the age of 16, and had planned her current pregnancy following a period of depression. Taylor was excluded from school for fighting and truancy in Year 9 (aged 13–14) and, after a period of non-attendance, continued her education in a pupil referral unit and then at a further education college, gaining two GCSEs. At the time of her first pregnancy, she was studying sports science at college:

> *Taylor:* I was doing sports science . . . I found out when I was pregnant them times. I wasn't really bothered about doing anything apart from being sick, being depressed and crying. So I never really, that never really followed through. That's it really.
> *Naomi:* So then you had the abortion, and then what did you do after that?
> *Taylor:* And then I just [pause] didn't really do nothing for two months, and then I went to back to . . . college, and I done a childcare course. I was there for like about two months. I was a bit depressed about the abortion, so learning about babies wasn't really my thing. You know what I'm saying? I wasn't really doing anything until I come here, I'm not even gonna lie. I weren't doing nothing.

Taylor was not unusual in having a fragmented educational path. Several of the young women interviewed had attended multiple educational settings between the ages of 11 and 18. However, Taylor found her time in the alternative educational scheme extremely valuable:

The tutors are friendly and they're supportive ... Everyone's just nice, everyone's funny. You get to see all the other previous girls, learners, and they bring their babies in ... You're just there to learn, and you're learning about something that's happening to *you*.

Taylor had decided to pursue sports science at college and wanted to be a physiotherapist, and did not see becoming a mother as a problem or a barrier to achieving this goal. When asked about her future plans she responded,

I just wanna do my course, finish my course, put my head down, and get my job. That's it. So I'm gonna work in sport physiotherapy ... My child knows when he sees me I'm gonna be his mum, as soon as he comes out he knows I'm his mum. But as a career, some people won't know me – if I don't get the job and I'm on the dole, the only person that'll know me is the Job Centre, if you understand where I'm coming from? So that's why you just better get your identity as a career, so that you can be a great mum and you can buy your child whatever you want ...

Like many of the other young women interviewed, Taylor perceived pregnancy as motivating her future aspirations. She also equated having a career with being a good mother, something that Reynolds (2005) found to be characteristic of the identities of Caribbean mothers.

For some of the young women, the qualifications achieved in the alternative educational scheme were the first they had gained in their lives – illuminating how, for some young women, becoming pregnant as a teenager leads to the kind of social and educational support that was lacking in mainstream educational settings.

Teenage years as the wrong time for childbearing?

As discussed earlier, teenage mothers are seen as deviating from the majority pattern of delaying motherhood until after entry into the labour market. The teenage years are characterized as the *wrong time* to have a baby. Teenage motherhood is seen as *ruining your life*, drawing attention to inappropriate sexual activity, bad/single parenting, and a culture of reliance on benefits. Jade, who is of White and Caribbean parentage and was aged 17 and pregnant at the time of interview, told a story of herself as a teenage 'bad girl' who had reformed and was now determined to 'make the best life for my child'. Jade had also been permanently excluded from school in Year 9 (age 13–14) and had attended a pupil referral unit. At the age of 15 she was arrested and charged with common assault and was under the supervision of a Youth Offending team for a year. She had spent some time in the care of the local authority but now had a good relationship with her parents. Jade describes herself as growing up 'too fast':

> My attitude was very, I grew up a bit too fast. When I was 13, I thought I was 16, so I thought I was, yeah, legal to have sex, and my boyfriend, he was a virgin himself, and I was more like, yeah, come on [laughs]. I started running away, from when I was like 13 to when I was 15. I hardly ever spent time at home coz I was always running away . . . Sex education-wise, I did it at school, but I didn't really pay much attention to it. I think I was in Year 6 [age 10–11] when I first got sex education, but it just shows you about the body and stuff, not about all the diseases you can get. But I was smart – I knew about it, because I always used to go to the [sexual health service] bus and get free condoms and all that nonsense.

Jade presents herself here as knowledgeable, independent and in control of her body, in spite of the instability of her home life during her early teenage years. She explains that she had not been using contraception with her boyfriend because a doctor had told her that she had 'low fertility'. After considering abortion, she decided to keep the baby. Jade reacted strongly against the idea of the prevention of teenage pregnancy, and that she would be categorized as a 'teenage parent':

> Back in the day you used to make kids my age marry and have babies, and now it's a bad thing. In a way, I see it as a advantage because by the time she's four, I could go to university or whatever I wanna do, and she's in school, she's in school from 9 till 3 and if there's after-school club, till 6 o'clock, so I could work and there's a lot of advantages there, but there's disadvantages as well . . . Some people generally want to have kids young . . . you can't prevent somebody, you cannot do it. And, why do they class it as just 'teenage pregnancy?' It's just somebody having a baby. Forget the teenage bit, coz in a couple of years they'll be an adult.

Although some of the young women equated pregnancy with growing up quickly, and giving up childish behaviour, others emphasized their maturity prior to pregnancy. Jade expresses her determination to be a good mother in terms of readiness for responsibility:

> When I was like 13, 14, I knew everyone, and I always had somewhere to go, and now, even before I was pregnant, I don't have

nowhere to go, or no one to see, because I'd already done it, I already lived that life of going raving and stuff ... But I just want the best for her ... Because I'm gonna have a child, it's making me think, if I'm not doing it for me, I have to do it for my child. I don't wanna be living on benefits for the rest of my life. I look at my mum ... she makes a good amount of money, has her own house with my dad, still together, and it's like I look at them and I think, why can't I do it? I can do it.

Teenage pregnancy as always a mistake?

It is often assumed that teenage conception is unplanned, so that pregnancy itself and the decision to keep the baby become a double mistake. While few admit to planning their pregnancies (see Cater and Coleman, 2006), there is a wide spectrum between a planned and an unplanned teenage pregnancy, with many young women reporting that, although they were not using any contraception, they were 'surprised' to be pregnant, or reporting that despite using contraception, they were not surprised to be pregnant. It is here that attention needs to be paid most closely to the 'logic of practice' that underpins the biography of the individual young woman. Samantha, a white young woman aged 18 and pregnant at the time of interview, had planned her pregnancy. Samantha was the second oldest of six children and had a difficult relationship with her family before leaving home. Like Jade, she emphasized her maturity and readiness for responsibility, citing a history of bulling at school and domestic conflict as putting her through 'more than teenagers go through'. Already disengaged from education, family problems resulted in Samantha dropping out of school in Year 11 (age 15–16) before she had taken her GCSEs. Since then, she had taken an E2E[3] course and achieved a childcare qualification at college and was proud of the way she had managed to get herself back on track after her mum kicked her out of the house:

> [I was] worrying about what am I gonna do next. Like you can't think about education in that time, you just think about what am I gonna do, I'm actually in a situation, like, and then once you get yourself back on your feet and you know, by the time I moved to the hostel I knew what I was gonna do, I knew I was going back to college and I knew what I was going to study. I've always wanted to be a teacher, so childcare was the only option at that time anyway, so I did childcare and I did work experience.

Like most of the other young women in the study, Samantha's idea of a future career had taken shape prior to pregnancy. She had been in a relationship with her boyfriend for five years, and described her decision to have a baby:

> It was planned. Obviously coz me and my boyfriend have been together for a long time, I trust him and stuff. Erm, I went to my GP and I told her in January, coz I got a flat and I was like, maybe it's time for me to tell her that I wanna get pregnant. And she gave me folic acid and she was like, take this, this is to protect the baby when you do get pregnant. And I found out I was pregnant in March.

Samantha's 'logic' is clear when put in the context of her familial and educational trajectory and her feelings of maturity. Like Taylor and Jade, she showed a determination to succeed in life and wanted the best for her child. Far from being a mistake, Samantha 'achieved' her pregnancy at a time that made sense to her. Far from lacking in aspirations, Taylor, Jade and Samantha had clear life goals that intertwined with and enhanced their mothering identities.

Conclusion

In this chapter, we have used qualitative evidence to describe and contest the meanings of teenage pregnancy. We began by revealing the very different place that sexual experience and parenthood hold in the imagined futures of young people growing up in contrasting social locations, suggesting the significance of the wider cultural and material context within which teenage pregnancy is given meaning. We then drew on qualitative research to show how the 'problem' of teenage motherhood is deeply personal for those involved. These young women do not consider early motherhood to be wrong or unusual. They work hard to counter prejudice informed by dominant discourses of the 'right' age or circumstances in which to become a mother. Paying attention to their narratives provides insight into their transition to motherhood and their changing identities and priorities at this critical moment in their lives. It is too easy to frame the lives and choices of disadvantaged groups in terms of lack (of aspiration, planning, self-esteem), and the policy framework of social exclusion can encourage a focus on such personal and cultural factors as explanations of material disadvantage. Yet qualitative evidence consistently points to the creativity and agency of young mothers as well as the very real material and personal challenges that they face (Lawlor and Shaw, 2002; Duncan, 2007). Rather than judging young mothers against the standard of an idealized norm of middle class, it may be that they are part of the range of family forms. As described by Judith Stacey (1998), these family forms only make sense as responses to new economic and social insecurities and the demise of the family wage.

Drawing policy messages from our chapter, we would point to the importance of recognizing young women's agency in the context of their social location, and the importance of motherhood within this. Ruth Levitas (2005) has argued that UK policy over the last decade has placed too much emphasis on employment as the sole route out of poverty, and that the channelling of teenage mothers into education, training or employment at the earliest opportunity represents an exclusion from mothering. Along with Alldred and David (2007), we suggest that the position of young women as *mothers* is being undermined by current policy. However, the value of some current provision for pregnant young women and mothers should not be overlooked. Some excellent models of educational provision and support for young mothers have flourished over the past decade. These models, as well as smaller post-16 interventions focusing on preparation for motherhood, social support and key skills, draw pregnant young women out of mainstream education but do so in a way that can provide vital attention to emotional and social needs. Yet such interventions are fragile and dependent on changing funding streams. For example, the alternative educational provision that Taylor, Jade and Samantha attended has been subject to significant disruption due to funding problems.

Notes

1. Sexual competence is defined in relation to four circumstantial variables: regret, willingness, autonomy and contraception use at first intercourse.
2. All names have been changed.
3. Entry to Employment (E2E) is a work-based programme for 16–18-year-olds not yet ready to enter further education, employment or an apprenticeship.

Acknowledgements

The authors would like to acknowledge Economic and Social Research Council funding of the research reported in this paper, including the Youth Values study (award number L129251020) and PhD studentship (award number PTA-031-2006-00238).

References

Alldred, P. and David, M. (2007) *Get Real About Sex: The Politics and Practice of Sex Education.* Maidenhead: Open University Press.

Arai, L. (2003) Low expectations, sexual attitudes and knowledge: explaining teenage pregnancy and fertility in English communities. Insights from qualitative research, *The Sociological Review*, 51(2): 199–217.

Barn, R. and Mantovani, N. (2007) Young mothers and the care system: contextualizing risk and vulnerability, *British Journal of Social Work*, 37: 225–43.

Berthoud, R. (2001) Teenage births to ethnic minority women, *Population Trends*, 104: 12–17.

Bourdieu, P. (1980) *The Logic of Practice*. Oxford: Blackwell.

Bradshaw, J., Finch, N. and Miles, J.N.V. (2005) Deprivation and variations in teenage conceptions and abortions in England, *Journal of Family Planning and Reproductive Health Care*, 31(1): 15–19.

Bynner, J., Elias, P., McKnight, A., Pan, H. and Pierre, G. (2002) *Young People's Changing Routes to Independence*. York: Joseph Rowntree Foundation.

Cater, S. and Coleman, L. (2006) *'Planned' Teenage Pregnancy: Perspectives of Young Parents from Disadvantaged Backgrounds*. Bristol: The Policy Press in associated with the Joseph Rowntree Foundation.

Cooke, J. and Owen J. (2007) 'A place of our own?': teenage mothers' views on housing needs and support models, *Children and Society*, 21: 56–68.

Dawson, N. and Hosie, A. (2005) *The Education of Pregnant Young Women and Young Mothers in England*. Bristol: University of Bristol.

Duncan, S. (2005) Mothering, class and rationality, *The Sociological Review*, 53(1): 50–76.

Duncan S. (2007) What's the problem with teenage parents? And what's the problem with policy? *Critical Social Policy*, 27(3): 307–34.

Ferri, E. and Smith, K. (2003) 'Partnership and parenthood' and 'family life', in E. Ferri, J. Bynner and M. Wadsworth (eds) *Changing Britain, Changing Lives: Three Generations at the Turn of the Century*. London: Institute of Education, Bedford Way Papers.

Furlong, A. and Cartmel, F. (2007) *Young People and Social Change: New Perspectives*. Maidenhead: Open University Press.

Graham, H. and McDermott, E. (2005) Qualitative research and the evidence base of policy: insights from studies of teenage mothers in the UK, *Journal of Social Policy*, 35(1): 21–37.

Henderson, S., Holland, J., McGrellis, S., Sharpe, S. and Thomson, R. (2007) *Inventing Adulthoods: A Biographical Approach to Youth Transitions*. London: SAGE.

Hirst, J., Formby, E. and Owen J. (2006) *Pathways into Parenthood: Reflections from Three Generations of Teenage Mothers and Fathers*. Sheffield: Sheffield Hallam University.

Hobcraft, J. and Kiernan, K. (2001) Childhood poverty, early motherhood and adult social exclusion, *British Journal of Sociology*, 52(3): 495–517.

Hosie, A. and Selman, P. (2006) Teenage pregnancy and social exclusion, in H.S. Holgate, R. Evans and F.K.O. Yuen (eds) *Teenage Pregnancy and Parenthood: Global Perspectives, Issues and Intervention*. London: Routledge.

Jones, G. (2005) The thinking and behaviour of young adults (aged 16–25), *Literature Review for the Social Exclusion Unit*, London: SEU.

Joshi, H. (2008) *Setting the Scene*, Presentation given at Modern Motherhood Conference, Family and Parenting Institute. London, 2 July 2008.

Kidger, J. (2004) Including young mothers: limitations to New Labour's strategy for supporting teenage parents, *Critical Social Policy*, 24(3): 291–311.

Lawlor, D. and Shaw, M. (2002) Too much too young? Teenage pregnancy is not a public health problem, *International Journal of Epidemiology*, 31: 552–4.

Lee, E., Clements, S., Ingham, R. and Stone, N. (2004) *A Matter of Choice? Explaining National Variations in Teenage Abortion and Motherhood*. York: Joseph Rowntree Foundation.

Letherby, G., Brown, G., DiMarco, H. and Wilson, C. (2002) *Pregnancy and Post-natal Experience of Young Women Who Become Pregnant under the Age of Twenty Years*. Final Report for Coventry Primary Care Trust. Coventry: Centre for Social Justice, Coventry University.

Levitas, R. (2005) *The Inclusive Society? Social Exclusion and New Labour*. Houndmills: Palgrave Macmillan.

MacDonald, R. and Marsh, J. (2005) *Disconnected Youth? Growing up in Britain's Poor Neighbourhoods*. Houndmills: Palgrave Macmillan.

McRobbie, A. (2004) Notes on postfeminism and popular culture: Bridget Jones and the new gender regime, in A. Harris (ed.) *All About the Girl: Culture, Power and Identity*. New York: Routledge.

Mitchell, W. and Green, E. (2002) 'I don't know what I'd do without our Mam': motherhood, identity and support networks, *The Sociological Review*, 50(1): 1–22.

Nilsen, A. (1999) Where is the future? Time and space as categories in analyses of young people's images of the future, *Innovation*, 12(2): 175–194.

Reynolds, T. (2005) *Caribbean Mothers: Identity and Experience in the UK*. London: The Tufnell Press.

Rudoe, N. (in press) *Young Motherhood, Social Exclusion and Educational Policy*. Unpublished PhD Thesis, The Open University.

Skeggs, B. (2004) *Class, Self, Culture*. London: Routledge.

Stacey, J. (1998) *Brave New Families: Stories of Domestic Upheaval in Late-twentieth-century America*. Berkeley, CA: University of California Press.

Thomson, R. (2000) Dream on: the logic of sexual practice, *Journal of Youth Studies*, 3(4): 407–27.

Thomson, R. and Kehily, M. J., with Hadfield, L. and Sharpe, S. (2008) *The Making of Modern Motherhood: Memories, Representations, Practices*. ESRC 'Identities and Social Action' programme final report. Available at http://www.open.ac.uk/socialsciences/identities/projects/Motherhood_brochure2008_ebook.pdf .

Tyler, I. (2008) 'Chav mum chav scum': class disgust in contemporary Britain, *Feminist Media Studies*, 8(1): 17–34.

United Nations Children's Fund (UNICEF) (2007) *Child Poverty in Perspective: An Overview of Child Well-being in Rich Countries*, Innocenti Report Card 7. Florence: Innocenti Research Centre.

Uren, Z., Sheers, D. and Dattani, N. (2007) Teenage conceptions by small area deprivation in England and Wales, 2001–2002, *Health Statistics Quarterly*, 33: 34–9.

Walkerdine, V., Lucey, H. and Melody, J. (2001) *Growing up Girl: Psychosocial Explorations of Gender and Class*. Houndmills: Palgrave Macmillan.

Wellings, K., Nanchahal, K., Macdowall, W. et al. (2001) Sexual behaviour in Britain: early heterosexual experience, *The Lancet*, 358: 1843–50.

Wellings, K., Wadsworth, J., Johnson, A., Field, J. and Macdowall, W. (1999) Teenage fertility and life chances, *Reviews of Reproduction*, 4(3): 184–90.

Wiggins, M., Oakley, A., Sawtell, M. et al. (2005) *Teenage Parenthood and Social Exclusion: A Multi-method Study: Summary Report of Findings*. London: Social Science Research Unit Report, Institute of Education.

Part 3

Health inequalities: understanding policy impacts

The impact of policies on socio-economic inequalities in health is a theme which runs through the chapters of the book. The theme is explicitly addressed in Part 3.

Two chapters – by Margaret Whitehead, Barbara Hanratty and Bo Burström and by Hilary Graham – discuss the distributive effects of social and economic policies, noting how policies can both widen and reduce inequalities in people's lives.

Margaret Whitehead, Barbara Hanratty and Bo Burström present evidence from cross-national and international studies of the impact of policies on socio-economic inequalities in long-term illnesses and disabilities. Their analysis highlights how governments can underwrite the living standards of poorer groups vulnerable both to long-term health conditions and to the downward drag that these conditions can exert on employment prospects and incomes.

Hilary Graham illustrates how policies can influence the unequal distribution of health determinants by focusing on two major determinants – household income and cigarette smoking. In the UK, as elsewhere, both display steep socio-economic gradients. Echoing the conclusions of earlier chapters, her analysis points to the critical role played by government policy in shaping both the overall level of health determinants within a society and their social distribution.

3.1 Unequal consequences of ill health: researching the role of public policy

Margaret Whitehead, Barbara Hanratty and Bo Burström

Introduction

There is an increasing focus in public policy around Europe on the challenge of tackling social inequalities in health, but before effective action can be developed, it is necessary to understand how the observed health inequalities are generated and maintained. What are the pathways to inequalities in health and where are the potential policy entry points along the way to tackle these inequalities? Do public policies themselves have differential impacts on different socio-economic groups in the population – and are the impacts negative or positive? This chapter focuses in particular on one of the potential pathways, relatively neglected in the past but gaining recognition more recently: the unequal consequences of ill health.

It begins by introducing the conceptual framework that encompasses unequal consequences of ill health, that is, how poor health may have different economic and social impacts for different socio-economic groups in society. It goes on to present three case studies to illustrate the various ways in which we have attempted to research the nature and extent of unequal consequences of ill health and to evaluate the impact of policy on these consequences. The first case study focuses on the exploitation of natural policy experiments to assess differential policy impacts, the second on the use of tracer diseases or conditions and the third on the value of longitudinal record linkage studies for identifying causal pathways. We discuss how unequal consequences may translate into further sickness in a downward spiral, contributing to the observed inequalities in health. The final section of the chapter considers the role of different types of policy in magnifying or preventing such adverse consequences, to address the question: what role for public policy?

Pathways to social inequalities in health: conceptual framework

We use Diderichsen's framework (Diderichsen et al., 2001) for mapping the impact of policies on the social pathways to health inequalities to help conceptualize the different mechanisms generating health inequalities and the possible policy entry points (Figure 3.1.1). In this framework, the pathways leading to ill health can be approached from the perspective of the individual or of society. The right-hand side of the figure considers an individual's social position and how that position influences exposure to important health risks such as poverty, nutritional deficiencies, health-damaging behaviours, dangerous working conditions and so on. Four main mechanisms are distinguished. The first is the process of *social stratification* which sorts the population into different social positions in a given society, thereby allocating different power and resources to different social positions (WHO CSDH, 2008). Groups that are better off typically have more power and opportunities to live a healthy life than groups

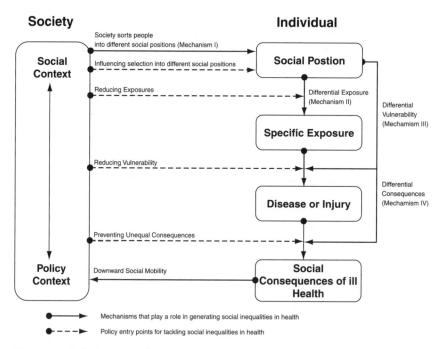

Figure 3.1.1 Framework for studying the pathways from the social context to health outcomes and for introducing policy interventions.
Source: adapted from Diderichsen et al. (2001), Figure 1.

that are less privileged (mechanism I). As discussed in Hilary Graham's introductry chapter, social position in itself is therefore considered to be an important determinant of social inequalities in health (Link and Phelan, 1996; Graham, 2007). This stratification is usually stronger when the social divisions in society are wider.

The second mechanism is *differential exposure*. Exposure to almost all risk factors (material, psycho-social and behavioural) is inversely related to social position – that is, the lower the social position, the greater the exposure to a variety of health hazards – and contributes to the generation of the familiar social gradient in health (mechanism II). Third, a specific exposure may or may not lead to ill health or disease for an individual, depending on whether other contributory risk factors or risk conditions are present and whether they combine together to produce a heightened effect (mechanism III: *differential vulnerability*). Fourth, the social and economic consequences of illness are not only dependent on the health problem suffered by the person, but also on the effects of the illness on the person's ability to stay employed, live independently and participate in their community. These effects may vary according to the social position of the individual (mechanism IV: *differential consequences* of disease). The social consequences of illness might also have a further impact on social stratification, for example, forcing a move to a lower-status job or unemployment, feeding back into the social and policy context (mechanism I again).

The left-hand side of the figure represents the societal perspective, focusing on how the prevailing social context interacts with and influences the individual pathways from social position to ill health. As part of the social context, policy may have an influence on the pathways between social position and health consequences at four distinct points represented in Figure 3.1.1:

- *Policy Entry Point A*: policy may influence the social position that individuals occupy in society. The education system and family policies, for example, may influence the opportunities people have to move up the social scale, and indeed, can influence how wide the gulf is between people in different social positions.
- *Policy Entry Point B:* policy may influence exposure to health hazards faced by people in different social positions. Many public health efforts that have been implemented so far to combat inequalities in health have been aimed at preventing people in disadvantaged positions from being exposed to poverty, unhealthy housing, dangerous working conditions, nutritional deficiencies and so on. These policies will often be designed to have a greater impact on more disadvantaged groups, thereby reducing the health gap.

- *Policy Entry Point C:* policy may influence the effect of being ex-posed to a hazardous factor. As noted under mechanism III, the size of the effect of a certain risk factor or risk condition will often be dependent on the presence of other contributory causes. For example, the impact on health of being poor or unemployed may vary across societies or even in different time periods within the same country. Local or national policies may be in place, for in-stance, which not only influence the risk of being poor (as in entry point B) but also either soften or reinforce the effects of being poor (entry point C).
- *Policy Entry Point D:* policies may influence the impact of being ill. Several types of policy, most prominently those concerned with the effectiveness and equity of healthcare services, may have a direct impact on morbidity and its consequences in terms of sur-vival, disability and daily living. The social consequences of being ill in a specific society may vary, and will partly depend on the way chronic illness interacts with a number of factors related to social context (for example, what state the local labour market is in and what policies are in place encouraging or discouraging people with disabilities or chronic conditions to have paid employment).

Researching mechanism IV: unequal consequences of ill health

In our research funded by the ESRC, MRC and Rockefeller Foundation, we set out to study the fourth mechanism in more depth: the differential so-cial and economic consequences of being sick. The following case studies illustrate the various ways we have attempted to research mechanism IV and the policy questions that it raises.

Case study 1: exploiting natural policy experiments on employment consequences

We have employed Anglo-Swedish comparative studies to investigate the differential impacts of public policies. The 2004 Wanless Report on future scenarios for public health called for the exploitation of 'natural policy experiments' to generate evidence from policies and practice currently being implemented (Wanless, 2003). The methodology for assessing the impact of such natural experiments in relation to health is still being re-fined, but cross-country comparative analysis has a promising part to play, especially for some of the major public policies that tend to be introduced nationwide, rather than in discreet 'intervention' and 'control' areas.

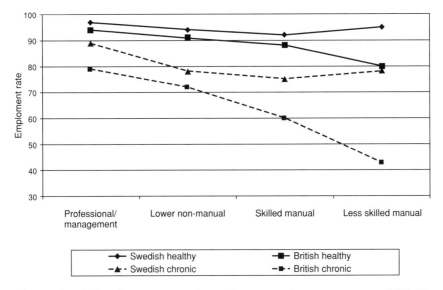

Figure 3.1.2 Employment rates by socio-economic group, men aged 25–59 with and without chronic illness, 1989–95.
Source: adapted from Burström et al. (2000) .

Taking advantage of the natural experiment provided by the very different labour market policies pursued in Britain and Sweden since the 1970s, we analysed the impact of chronic illness on employment for men and women in the two countries and in different socio-economic groups. We employed secondary data analysis of household survey data, the British *General Household Survey* (GHS) and the Swedish *Survey of Living Conditions* (ULF), from nationally representative annual samples over two decades. At the start of the project, great care was taken to find and create comparable variables for analysis. Data for several years were combined to increase the sample size in some of the sub-groups we wished to study.

Figures 3.1.2. and 3.1.3 illustrate both the adverse employment consequences of having a chronic illness and the social gradient in those consequences. For both men and women, not only did having a chronic illness reduce the chances of being in paid employment, but, crucially, the impact varied by socio-economic group and by country. Figure 3.1.2 shows very little difference in employment rates in Sweden compared to Britain for healthy men in the three professional/managerial, lower non-manual and skilled manual groups. Only among the fourth group – less skilled manual – is there a marked difference between the two countries, with a much lower employment rate among healthy less skilled manual men in British than in Sweden. Among men with a chronic illness, however, British men

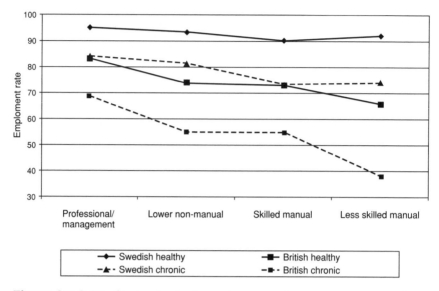

Figure 3.1.3 Employment rates by socio-economic group, women aged 25–59 with and without chronic illness, 1989–95.
Source: adapted from Burström et al. (2003).

in each socio-economic group not only fare much worse than Swedish men with chronic illness in their equivalent group, but also the decline in employment with decreasing socio-economic group is very steep in Britain; much less so in Sweden. Figure 3.1.3 shows the employment pattern among women in the two countries, revealing much lower employment rates for British healthy women in each socio-economic group compared with Swedish healthy women, in contrast to the much smaller differences found among healthy men in the two countries. Among chronically ill women, the marked stepwise decline in employment from professional to less skilled manual women in Britain, but not in Sweden, mirrors the pattern found for men.

We were able to set these patterns in a broader context by looking at social gradients in employment among people with chronic illness over time, from the early 1980s to the late 1990s. The social gradient in employment among people with chronic illness was pronounced in Britain for both men and women and became steeper over time. For example, employment rates ranged from 44 per cent for unskilled manual women to 64 per cent for professional women in the first half of the 1980s and widened further, so that by the 1990s the employment rates had declined to 38 per cent for unskilled manual while increasing to 69 per cent for professional women (Burström et al., 2003). An even stronger social gradient was evident for British men, among whom employment rates ranged from 56 per cent for unskilled manual men to 88 per cent for professional men in the 1980s, and from 43 per cent to 79 per cent in the 1990s (Burström et al., 2000).

We found a very different pattern for Sweden. There was no clear social gradient in employment in the 1980s for women with chronic illness, but a divide between manual and non-manual women emerged by the 1990s, a trend that was not evident among healthy Swedish women (Burström et al., 2003). Among Swedish men, there was a shallow gradient in employment, ranging from 82 per cent for unskilled manual men to 92 per cent for professional men in the 1980s, and no real difference in employment rates among three socio-economic groups in the 1990s, only a split between the professionals, with a rate of 89 per cent and the remaining three groups with rates between 75–8 per cent (Burström et al., 2000). Overall, having chronic illness had much more severe consequences for the employment chances of both men and women in Britain compared with Sweden.

Case study 2: using tracer conditions to explore differential consequences

One problem in using a general indicator of ill health, such as limiting long-standing illness, to study consequences is that the impact of being sick is likely to vary, sometimes markedly, depending on the type of health problem or disease that a person has. Some conditions cause minor disruption to daily life, while others have a major influence on ability to work and live independently; some are relatively cheap to treat and can be handled in primary care, while others require very expensive procedures and specialist treatment away from home. In an attempt to achieve a closer comparison of like with like, we have been selecting specific diagnoses as 'tracer conditions', to compare and contrast the consequences of having such a diagnosis for different groups in the population, including how employment chances vary and whether there is differential access to services for the care that the patients actually need for their particular health problem.

First, taking advantage of linked diagnostic and socio-economic data for the entire population of Stockholm County, we explored the employment consequences over five years subsequent to hospital admission of having a diagnosed musculoskeletal disorder, such as arthritis or back problems, among two groups of patients (Holland et al., 2006). Patients who were in employment at baseline had an increased risk of subsequently leaving the labour market relative to people in paid work who did not have musculoskeletal disorders. Manual workers with musculoskeletal disorders

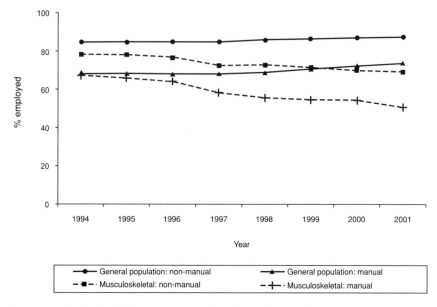

Figure 3.1.4 Trends in age-standardized employment rates among patients who received hospital inpatient care in 1996 for a musculoskeletal disorder and among the general population, manual and non-manual occupational classes, residents of Stockholm County, Sweden, aged 31–64.
Source: adapted from Holland et al. (2006), Figure 2.

left the labour market at a faster rate than their manual peers in the general population after hospitalization in 1996. Indeed, there was a slight increase in employment rates after 1998 for manual workers in the general population, while rates continued to decline for manual workers with musculoskeletal disorders. A similar, though less marked, decline in employment was seen for non-manual workers with musculoskeletal disorders, while non-manual workers in the general population maintained a high, and steady, level of employment. In a further analysis, we calculated age-standardized employment rates for *all* patients with a diagnosed musculoskeletal disorder, regardless of their employment status at baseline, and this revealed widening inequality during 1996–2001 between the employment rates of people with a musculoskeletal disorder and those of the general population. Furthermore, while employment rates rose in the general population of Stockholm County during this period, they fell among patients with musculoskeletal disorders (Figure 3.1.4).

Second, we have studied financial consequences and impact on access to appropriate care for specific diseases in countries which have undergone major health system reforms as a way of testing the impact of the health

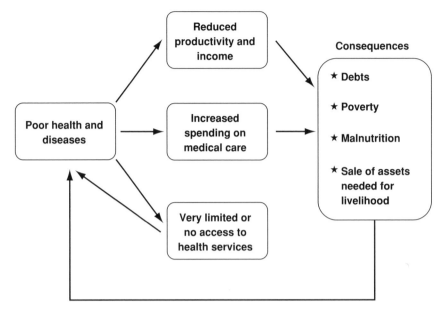

Figure 3.1.5 Linkages between poor health and poverty.
Source: adapted from Dahlgren and Whitehead (2007), Figure 2.1.

and social protection system. The possible linkages between poor health and poverty in such countries are depicted in Figure 3.1.5 and include falling into debt, impoverishment, malnutrition, untreated sickness and sale of assets needed for livelihood, feeding back into further damage to health in a downward spiral (Whitehead, et al., 2001; McIntyre et al., 2006).

In China, for example, we focused on tuberculosis (TB) symptoms. We used TB symptoms as a 'tracer condition' to investigate receipt of appropriate care and affordability for different socio-economic groups of rural residents. We carried out secondary data analysis of the Chinese *National Health Survey* for 2003, which included 40,000 rural households containing over 143,000 individuals, 2300 of whom were identified as having symptoms of TB. Of these people with TB symptoms, over a third did not seek any professional care, with low-income groups less likely to seek care than more affluent counterparts. Of those seeking care, only a third received any of the recommended diagnostic tests. Of the 182 patients with a confirmed TB diagnosis, just over half received treatment at the recommended level. Treatment was less likely to be received by people lacking health insurance or material assets. Our study illustrated the severe financial consequences of having TB symptoms or being a diagnosed

TB patient in rural China. The total annual medical expenses of people with TB symptoms with low income was equivalent to over 45 per cent of total annual household income for a low-income household. Even for the high-income households, the costs amounted to over 16 per cent of annual household income in that income bracket (Zhang et al., 2007). The financial burden was even greater for diagnosed TB patients in this study. Given that out-of-pocket medical payments of over 10 per cent of annual household income are defined as 'catastrophic' in World Bank analyses (Xu et al., 2003), the level of payments of people with TB symptoms and of diagnosed patients in our study would almost certainly be impoverishing. Added to this, the third of people with TB symptoms who did not seek any professional care, many citing cost as a barrier, would contain people who would go on to develop TB, which, without treatment, would lead to further deterioration in health, with knock-on effects on ability to work and earn a living. Hence, health care costs could have serious consequences for the individual, as well as for the health of the population.

In Sri Lanka, we have used qualitative interviews with patients diagnosed with specific diseases to understand more about the social and economic consequences of having those diseases in the specific policy context (Perera, Gunatilleke and Bird, 2007; Perera, Whitehead et al., 2007). One of the diseases we looked at was lymphatic filariasis (LF), a parasitic disease caused by microscopic, thread-like worms which live in the human lymph system and are spread by mosquitoes. While rarely fatal, LF can cause chronic suffering, disability, and social stigma. It can lead to swollen limbs – a condition known as filarial lymphoedema or filarial elephantiasis – and, in men, to swelling of the scrotum (filarial hydrocele). We used purposive sampling to select 60 men and women with filarial lymphoedema (45 with filarial elephantiasis and 15 men with filarial hydrocele) from the south of Sri Lanka in 2004–5. Participants were selected to give a balance of men and women, poor and non-poor and a range of stages of the disease. Their experiences and consequences of the disease for the household were explored with in-depth qualitative, semi-structured interviews. LF was extremely debilitating over a long period of time. The social isolation from stigma caused emotional distress and delayed diagnosis and treatment, resulting in undue advancement of the disease. Free treatment services at government clinics were avoided because the participants' condition would be identifiable in public. Loss of income because of the condition was reported by all households in the sample, not just confined to the poorest. Households that were already on low income, however, were pushed into near destitution by LF, from which it was almost impossible to escape. Low-income households also had less opportunity to obtain effective treatment from distant clinics, and had living and working conditions that made hygiene and compliance more difficult. It was clear from this study that this highly vulnerable category of patients had low visibility, and had become marginalized and forgotten. One important conclusion was that, with an estimated 300,000 cases of elephantiasis, and around 300,000 men with filarial hydrocele, the afflicted households would need help and support for many years to come. They should not be neglected, but be specially targeted to identify, reach and care for them (Perera, Whitehead et al., 2007).

Case study 3: using longitudinal record linkages to trace sequence of events

The study of unequal health consequences requires information on events over time, and there are a number of sources of relevant data available to researchers. Life-course epidemiologists, for example, have made a major contribution to the understanding of inequalities in health by analysing data from UK longitudinal studies such as the Whitehall Study (Marmot and Brunner, 2005) and the national birth cohorts (see Chapters 1.1 and 1.2). Although rich sources of information, cohort studies are expensive to conduct, and they are inevitably defined by the way in which the sample is selected, and the data the investigators decided to collect at the outset. To avoid some of these limitations, in our research we have exploited the value of longitudinal, linked datasets in Sweden. Offering high-quality information covering whole populations, these administrative resources contain data on births and deaths, health service utilization, income and welfare benefits for individuals that allow us to examine social patterning of outcomes over time. In this case study, we consider the time leading up to death.

Many people have more contact with health services in their final year than at any other time in their lives, and the care required can be intensive and costly. It has been estimated that as much as one-third of life-time health care expenditure occurs in the final year (Hogan et al., 2001). The high cost of services in the last year of life gives health care providers a strong motive to ensure they collect relevant data about their services. Although findings from time-to-death cost analyses are not entirely consistent across different health systems, approaching death does appear to be associated with increased health service expenditure, with population ageing simply delaying the years of high spending to the end of life, in some cases with a small shift away from acute care costs (Payne et al., 2007). The end of life may also be a time of financial stress for patients and caregivers, as well as for health providers. Illness may increase household expenses directly with the costs of travel and medicines, or indirectly by limiting the amount of paid work that can be done by the patient or carers. As with any financial pressures, the poorest in society are likely to be the most severely affected. At the same time, the accumulated effects of living with disadvantage over a lifetime leave poorer people experiencing greater severity of illness, more co-morbidities and in many cases, death at younger ages (see Chapter 1.2). Hence, the last year of life is a particularly important area of study for inequalities researchers. We should expect an equitable welfare system to be providing a greater amount of care for people from lower socio-economic groups, to match their greater health needs. With their focus on costs and cost savings, governments, local authorities and health services have data that could be used to examine their own performance, and review how equitable their services really are. The following are two examples of such analyses.

In the first example, we analysed Swedish data to identify which social groups are most vulnerable to financial and welfare policies at the end of life, by investigating absolute and relative movement in income in the three years leading up to death (Hanratty, Burström, Walander et al., 2007). The rationale for this study was that illness may result in downward social mobility, and that loss of a spouse may have devastating financial and social consequences for the survivor. The way in which financial circumstances change in the years before a death may also have important consequences for the individual's ability to cope with the illness, and their eligibility for welfare benefits. High-quality income data from tax registers were available for 14,221 of the 16,617 adults who died in Stockholm County in 2002. We found that the greatest changes in income were experienced by the poorest groups, who had both the highest percentage increases and decreases in income of all the decedents. As the worst off are least likely to have savings or insurance, some of the increases in their absolute incomes are likely to be due to supportive Swedish social welfare policies. Conversely, the highest percentage decreases in income among the poorest groups indicate that the long-standing policies were still not protecting everyone in the population (Hanratty, Burström, Walander et al. 2007).

In the second example, we used individual-level data on the entire population of Stockholm County Council (1.8 million) to investigate whether public expenditure on health care in Stockholm County in the 12 months before death varied with the socio-economic status of the patient (Hanratty, Burström, Möller et al., 2007). We found that county council expenditure on health care in the last year of life rose with increasing income of the decedent. The total age-standardized spend increased by 60 per cent across the five income groups. People with higher incomes were recipients of higher public spending on health care, taking into account differences in age, sex and major diagnoses (Hanratty, Burström, Möller et al., 2007).

The health inequalities literature predicts that people with lower incomes will, on average, have greater health needs, so they should require more public spending when they become patients. Our contradictory findings may result from systematic variation in the incidence of expensive-to-treat diseases across income groups, but we believe that it is more likely that affluent, better educated patients and their families were negotiating more costly care. This could have taken the form of extra tests or treatments, or it is possible that they were obtaining care in more expensive facilities. Unit costs in a teaching hospital, for example, may be higher than care in a less prestigious centre. Although these hypotheses could not be tested further with the existing datasets, the results stimulated politicians and health administrators in Stockholm County to set up a task force to look specifically at the services they are providing and whether the system was operating in an inequitable way (Hanratty, Burström, Möller et al., 2007).

Conclusion: what role for public policy?

Public policy may contribute to both the creation and amelioration of the adverse consequences of ill health uncovered in the studies above. Three main policy areas are relevant to this discussion, operating at policy entry point D of Figure 3.1.1: income maintenance policies, labour market policies to promote the employment of chronically ill or disabled people, and vocational rehabilitation to tackle ill health and thereby increase the chances of getting a job.

First there are income-maintenance policies, which seek to maintain income when people fall sick and their income would otherwise drop if they could no longer work (Diderichsen, 2002). Long-term poverty among families is particularly damaging to health as it has far-reaching effects on prerequisites for the healthy development of children, such as good nutrition, housing and education (see Chapter 1.1). It is more damaging than shorter periods or occasional episodes of poverty (Benzeval and Judge, 2001). The avoidance of long-term poverty when people become unemployed or fall sick has therefore been one of the motivating forces behind the development of income-maintenance policies in modern welfare systems. These policies may, however, have differential effects on different social groups in the population, depending on how they are organized. In some circumstances, they may have the paradoxical effect of mitigating poverty across the population while at the same time widening inequalities, including health inequalities.

Our studies of income changes in Sweden in the last three years of life illustrate the importance of monitoring for differential effects of policies. The results show that absolute income levels were maintained in all

20 income groups but that, in relative terms, three-quarters moved into a lower income group during their final three years of life. Changes in absolute and relative income have different implications. All groups experienced small increases in household income in absolute terms in the three years before death. This could be predicted by increasing age and inflation. In relative terms, however, the greatest changes in income were experienced by the poorest groups, who had both the highest percentage increases and decreases in income of all the decedents. This suggests that some aspects of Swedish social welfare policies are working well in terms of making income transfers that benefit the poorest the most but still fall short of preventing income decline for all groups, especially the poorest. This is all the more surprising as Sweden has one of the most generous welfare systems in the world in terms of support for the sick (Fritzell and Lundberg, 2005). Equally revealing was the finding from our analyses of the *British Household Panel Survey* of people in the last year of life, which found financial strain was common among decedents aged over 65 in Britain, but fewer than 1 in 7 of those who were under financial strain were receiving an illness-related benefit, even though many should have been eligible to receive financial help (Hanratty et al., 2008)

Second, labour market policies may promote or hinder the chances of people with chronic illness or disability getting and keeping jobs, and thereby maintaining a decent standard of living. How well people with chronic illness fare in the labour market depends on several factors, including macro-economic developments but also on labour and social policy measures which may vary between countries. The value of taking advantage of cross-country natural policy experiments is illustrated by Anglo-Swedish studies. Sweden has one of the most regulated labour markets in Europe, Britain one of the least regulated. In addition, Sweden has launched active retraining and rehabilitation programmes to help unemployed people with chronic illnesses get back to work, as part of its commitment to state support and welfare provision. Two contrasting hypotheses have been formulated in this context:

- that the more flexible, deregulated labour market in Britain would result in higher employment rates than in Sweden, for those with and without limiting long-standing illness;
- that, because of active labour market measures and associated policies, people with limiting long-standing illness would have a stronger attachment to the labour market in Sweden than in Britain, even during periods of reduced demand for labour.

These hypotheses were explored in the studies outlined in Case study 1 (Burström et al., 2000, 2003). The findings indicate that, while Britain has adopted policies since the early 1980s to deregulate the labour market,

Sweden, in contrast, had developed strong employment security policies. The impact of these contrasting policies was revealed when analysing how well people with chronic illness fare in the labour markets of the two countries. Contrary to the hypothesis that groups with fewer skills and limiting illness should be more easily employed on a deregulated labour market, these groups fared worse in Britain than in Sweden. Furthermore, the inequalities between different socio-economic groups in the social consequences of chronic illness were much smaller in Sweden than in Britain. These studies, therefore, lend no support to the first hypothesis. There would appear to be no benefit for Sweden in copying British deregulation policies in terms of opportunities for people with chronic illness to get and to keep jobs.

Third, vocational and medical rehabilitation could potentially play an important role in improving the quality of life of chronically ill or disabled people and in helping them become fit enough to return to paid employment. We asked: what had the Swedish policy experiments on rehabilitation to offer in terms of lessons for Britain and other countries? Evaluations of the Swedish efforts to increase employment among those with limiting long-term illness during the 1990s indicate that these experiments failed when the effects were measured in employment rates. These programmes were however conceived in a situation (1990) when labour was in short supply and the high rates of sickness absence were more a result of high employment rates among the ill, rather than ineffective rehabilitation. By the time the programmes were implemented, demand for labour had collapsed and competition for the jobs had sharpened. Hardly surprising then, that the powerful macro-economic changes swamped any effects of improved medical and vocational rehabilitation. Hence, the Swedish experiments in rehabilitation are not likely to account for the differences between Britain and Sweden observed in our empirical study in relation to employment, unemployment and economic inactivity among people with chronic illness. The underlying employment protection legislation and traditional political commitment to full employment in Sweden are more likely candidates to explain the higher rates of employment among these sections of the population.

Overall, we have found compelling evidence of the wider consequences of ill health and how they differ, depending on social position and on policy context. Our overarching conclusion from these studies is that public policy has a pivotal role to play in addressing these unequal consequences of ill health. The possibility of adverse effects should not, however, be overlooked. Above all, there is a pressing need to uncover differential impacts of public policies and to understand much more about the context in which the polices are played out, to be able to devise more effective action.

Acknowledgements

This research was supported by the Medical Research Council Health of the Public Fellowship (Barbara Hanratty); joint Anglo-Swedish funding from the Economic and Social Research Council, Swedish Council for Working Life and Social Research and Stockholm County Council (Bo Burström and Margaret Whitehead) and studies in China and Sri Lanka by the Rockefeller Foundation (Margaret Whitehead). The authors alone bear the responsibility for the analyses and interpretations presented here.

References

Benzeval, M. and Judge, K. (2001) Income and health: the time dimension, *Social Science and Medicine*, 52: 1371–90.

Burström, B., Whitehead, M., Lindholm, C. and Diderichsen, F. (2000) Inequality in the social consequences of illness: how well do people with long-term illness fare in the British and Swedish labor markets? *International Journal of Health Services*, 30(3): 435–51.

Burström, B., Holland, P., Diderichsen, F. and Whitehead, M. (2003) Winners and losers in flexible labour markets: the fate of women with chronic illness in contrasting policy environments, *International Journal of Health Services*, 33(2): 199–207.

Dahlgren, G. and Whitehead, M. (2007) *European Strategies for Tackling Social Inequities in Health: Levelling up Part 2.* Copenhagen: WHO. Available at: http://www. euro. who.int/socialdeterminants/publications/ publications

Diderichsen, F. (2002) Income maintenance policies: determining their potential impact on socio-economic inequalities in health, in J. Mackenbach and M. Bakker (eds) *Reducing Inequalities in Health: A European Perspective*. London: Routledge.

Diderichsen F., Evans T. and Whitehead M. (2001) The social basis of disparities in health, in T. Evans, M. Whitehead, F. Diderichsen, A. Bhuiya and M. Wirth (eds) *Challenging Inequities in Health: From Ethics to Action*. New York: Oxford University Press.

Fritzell, J. and Lundberg, O. (2005) Fighting inequalities in health and income: one important road to welfare and social development, in O. Kangas and J. Palme (eds) *Social Policy and Economic Development in the Nordic Countries*. Basingstoke: Palgrave Macmillan.

Graham, H. (2007) *Unequal Lives: Health and Socio-economic Inequalities*. Maidenhead: Open University Press.

Hanratty, B., Burström, B., Möller, I. and Whitehead, M. (2007) Inequality in the face of death? A record linkage study of public expenditure on healthcare for different socio-economic groups in the last year of life, *Journal of Health Services Research and Policy*, 12(2): 90–4.

Hanratty, B., Burström, B., Walander, A. and Whitehead, M. (2007) Changes in income in the years before death: a record linkage study in Stockholm county, *Journal of Epidemiology and Community Health*, 61(5): 447–8.

Hanratty, B., Jacoby, A. and Whitehead, M. (2008) Socio-economic differences in service use, payment and receipt of illness-related benefits in the last year of life: findings from the British Household Panel Survey, *Palliative Medicine*, 22: 248–55.

Hogan, C., Lunney, J., Gabel, J. and Lynn, J. (2001) Medicare beneficiaries' costs of care in the last year of life, *Health Affairs* (Millwood), 20: 188–95.

Holland, P., Burström, B., Möller, I. and Whitehead, M. (2006) Gender and socio-economic variations in employment among patients with a diagnosed musculoskeletal disorder: a longitudinal record linkage study in Sweden, *Rheumatology*, 45: 1016–22.

Link, B.G. and Phelan, J. (1996) Understanding sociodemographic differences in health: the role of fundamental social causes, *American Journal of Public Health*, 86(4): 471–3.

McIntyre, D., Thiede, M., Dahlgren, G. and Whitehead, M. (2006) What are the economic consequences for households of illness and paying for health care in low- and middle-income country contexts? *Social Science and Medicine*, 62: 858–65.

Marmot, M. and Brunner, E. (2005) Cohort profile: the Whitehall II study, *International Journal of Epidemiology*, 34: 251–6.

Payne, G., Laporte, A., Deber, R. and Coyte, P.C. (2007) Counting backwards to health care's future: using time-to-death modelling to identify changes in end-of-life morbidity and the impact of aging on health care expenditures, *The Milbank Quarterly*, 85(2): 213–57.

Perera, M., Gunatilleke, G. and Bird, P. (2007) Falling into the medical poverty trap in Sri Lanka: what can be done? *International Journal of Health Services*, 37(2): 379–98.

Perera, M., Whitehead, M., Molyneux, D., Weerasooriya, M. and Gunatilleke, G. (2007) Neglected patients in a neglected disease? Qualitative study of Lymphatic Filariasis, *PLOS Neglected Tropical Diseases*, 1(2): e128.

UCL Department of Epidemiology and Public Health (2008) *The Whitehall II Study*. Available at: http://www.ucl.ac.uk/whitehallII/index.htm.

Wanless, D. (2003) *Securing Good Health for the Whole Population: Population Health Trend*. London: HMSO.

Whitehead, M., Dahlgren, G. and Evans, T. (2001) Equity and health sector reforms: can low-income countries escape the medical poverty trap? *The Lancet*, 358: 833–6.

World Health Organization (WHO) Commission on Social Determinants of Health (CSDH) (2008) *Closing the Gap in a Generation*. Final report of the Commission on Social Determinants of Health. Geneva: WHO.

Xu, K., Evans, D.B., Kawabata, K. et al. (2003) Household catastrophic health expenditure: a multi-country analysis, *The Lancet*, 362(9378): 111–17.

Zhang. T., Tang, S., Jun, G. and Whitehead, M. (2007) Persistent problems of access to appropriate, affordable TB services in rural China: experiences of different socio-economic groups, *BMC Public Health*, 7: 19.

3.2 Tackling health inequalities: the scope for policy

Hilary Graham

Introduction

The last decade has seen major changes in public health policy. New strategies are combining the traditional focus on improving population health with a commitment to reducing health inequalities. The strategies identify tackling the determinants of health as a way of advancing both goals together. However, how a determinants-oriented approach can achieve both better overall health and greater health equity is often skated over. What this requires are policies that not only improve access to health determinants for the population as a whole; they must also address the unequal distribution of health determinants between socio-economic groups.

The chapter is set against this backcloth. It begins by discussing the new health strategies before exploring how policies can influence the distribution of health determinants. It focuses on two key determinants highlighted in earlier chapters: socio-economic circumstances and health behaviour. As these chapters have noted, it is the persistence of inequalities in people's circumstances that underlies the persistence of socio-economic inequalities in health: this chapter focuses on household income as one core dimension of people's socio-economic position. Health behaviour has been identified as the primary mechanism linking wider determinants like socio-economic position to the leading causes of death in high-income countries and, increasingly, across the world (Lopez et al., 2006). Among the behavioural risk factors, health-damaging diets, physical inactivity and cigarette smoking have been singled out (Beaglehole and Magnus, 2002). The chapter takes cigarette smoking as its behavioural example. It is one which exemplifies many of the challenges facing public health policy in the 21st century.

A new approach to public health

Over the last 10 years, a raft of new public health strategies has been launched in high-income countries. They are distinguished by an emphasis on tackling health inequalities and tackling fundamental determinants.

First, the goals of public health policy have been reconfigured to include both improving overall health and reducing inequalities in its distribution. Thus in England – as in Northern Ireland, Scotland and Wales – the twin goals are 'improving health for all and tackling health inequality' (SSH, 1999: 5). Similarly, the US strategy 'is designed to achieve two overarching goals: increase quality and years of healthy life (and) eliminate health disparities' (USDHHS, 2000: 2); in Canada, 'the goals of the Strategy are to improve overall health outcomes and reduce health disparities' (ACPHHS, 2005: 10). Sweden's public health strategy fuses these goals into a single vision for public health: 'to achieve good health on equal terms' (MHSA, 2000: 11). Norway goes further, noting that the goal is 'not to further improve the health of the people that already enjoy good health' but 'now is to bring the rest of the population up to the same level as the people who have the best health – levelling up' (NMHCS, 2007: 5).

At global level, too, tackling health inequalities has moved up the policy agenda, with the World Health Organization (WHO, 2005: 4) committing its member states to 'tackle poor health and inequalities as a matter of urgency'. Goals have been set for Europe, with improving health placed alongside reducing 'the health gap between socio-economic groups within countries . . . by substantially improving the level of health of disadvantaged groups' (WHO Europe, 1999: 3, 16). The WHO Commission on Social Determinants of Health (CSDH) has endorsed an equity-oriented approach to public health, urging international agencies and national governments 'to close the health gap in a generation' (WHO CSDH, 2008: 197).

Second, strategies launched over the last decade share an emphasis on what are called 'wider determinants' and 'underlying causes' of health. For example, Scotland's policy blueprint argues that 'a fresh approach is necessary – a public health strategy which addresses the root causes of our health problems' (SSS, 1998: 1). It is a theme reiterated elsewhere in the UK, where again governments claim to be 'addressing the underlying determinants of health – dealing with the underlying causes of health inequalities' (DH, 2003: 5). Beyond the UK, the new strategies speak of 'tackling broader determinants' (New Zealand: MH, 2000: 5) and setting objectives for 'health determinants' (Sweden: Ågren, 2003: 5). At international level, too, the emphasis is on tackling 'basic determinants' and 'root causes of socio-economic inequities' (WHO Europe 1999: 4).

Terms like 'basic determinants' and 'root causes' cover a range of social influences on people's health. For some, they include the political and economic structures which produce inequalities in people's lives. For example, the CSDH regards the major determinants of health not as 'the immediate causes of disease' like high blood pressure or cigarette smoking, but as 'the "causes of the causes" – the fundamental global and national structures of the social hierarchy and the socially determined conditions these create in which people grow, live, work, and age' (WHO CSDH, 2008: 42). Its emphasis on hierarchical structures is unusual, however. Most policy documents employ a more downstream concept of basic determinants. Living and working conditions are often included. For example, the strategy documents in England and Canada note that the term includes 'determinants of health such as the work environment, housing and living conditions' (DH, 2001: 16) and 'the living and working environments that affect people's health, (and) the conditions that enable and support people in making healthy choices' (ACPHHS, 2005: 10). These determinants are seen to influence health both directly and through health behaviours. In consequence, health behaviours are often identified as a wider determinant. For example, the US strategy includes lifestyle factors like smoking among 'the array of critical influences that determine the health of individuals and communities' (USDHHS, 2000: 18).

Whether the emphasis is on social conditions or health behaviours, the policy blueprints are clear that tackling wider determinants is essential if the twin goals of overall health gain and greater health equity are to be advanced. However, it is often less clear what this means. Few strategy documents spell out that it requires policies which improve overall access to the determinants of health *and* level-up access to health determinants across socio-economic groups. For example, it requires both improvements in average living standards *and* a greater improvement in the living standards of poorer groups; it requires both reductions in overall rates of cigarette smoking *and* a faster rate of decline among more disadvantaged groups. What matters for health equity is therefore tackling the unequal distribution of health determinants (Graham, 2004; Graham and Kelly, 2004). Improving the poor health of poor groups and flattening the broader social gradient in health turns on governments addressing what the CSDH calls the 'unequal distribution of health-damaging experiences' (WHO CSDH, 2008: 1).

The chapter focuses on two health determinants to examine how policies can do this. It looks at inequalities in people's socio-economic circumstances, taking household income as its measure of people's circumstances, and at inequalities in health behaviour, taking cigarette smoking as its example. For each determinant, the sections provide some historical background before considering the role that governments can play in tackling the unequal distribution of health determinants.

Inequalities in socio-economic circumstances: the scope for policy

Until the 20th century, governments in most high-income countries played only a minimal role in promoting the welfare of their populations. They were generally reluctant to intervene in the workings of the market economy and there was little publicly funded welfare provision, either in cash (like unemployment benefits and state pensions) or in kind (like health care and education). But the 20th century saw a marked increase in state regulation of the labour market and in the provision of welfare benefits and services across high-income countries.[1] This trend was particularly marked from the 1950s to the 1970s. By the end of the 1970s, social expenditure – devoted principally to income-maintenance programmes to support people during illness, unemployment and old age, together with health care, education and housing – had risen to 25 per cent of GDP in the UK. Elsewhere in Europe, welfare spending was higher still, reaching over 33 per cent of GDP in Denmark, Sweden and The Netherlands (Therborn, 1989). Even in the USA, social spending increased markedly, climbing to 20 per cent of GDP by 1980 (Amenta and Skocpol, 1989). Then as now, welfare spending was funded by taxation in various forms. This includes direct taxes on earnings and investments, indirect taxes on goods and services, and payroll taxes paid by workers and employers.

Collective systems for funding and meeting people's needs have major redistributive effects. Most notably, they distribute resources across people's lives (Falkingham and Hills, 1995). They protect living standards and meet welfare needs at periods in the life course when individuals are most vulnerable by transferring resources from periods where they are earning and in good health. The transfer process works by collecting funds from working-age adults in the form of taxes, and paying them out in the form of cash benefits and welfare services to the non-working generations. Thus, taxes and benefits spread out income between childhood (when the individual is too young to work and pay tax), adulthood (when they are likely to be doing both), and older age (when they are retired). Welfare services, too, have a strong life-course orientation, with governments spending most on younger and older age groups. The largest budgets are for education and health care, and, in all welfare systems, children are the major users of education and older people are the major consumers of health care (Ginsberg, 1993; Sefton, 2002).

Welfare systems also redistribute resources between households. They therefore provide governments with levers through which to level up

resources between socio-economic groups. For example, educational inequalities can be reduced by equalizing access to education through free
and universal provision, and inequalities in working conditions can be
tackled by setting minimum wage levels and strengthening safety standards and employment rights for low-paid workers. Capturing the impacts of such policies is not easy. While still complex, policy impacts on
inequalities in incomes are more straightforward to measure. Household
income is therefore often taken as the metric through which to assess
the redistributive effects of government policy. For these assessments, inequalities in household income are measured 'before policy' and 'after
policy'.

To inform their analyses, researchers make a distinction between 'market income' and 'disposable income'. Market income is income received
from earnings, pensions, shares and property, before taxes are deducted
and cash benefits are received. It therefore provides a measure of 'pre-
policy' inequalities. Disposable income is income after government intervention through direct taxation and cash transfers: it therefore provides a
measure of 'post-policy' inequalities. Using this information, researchers
have undertaken two types of analysis. The first takes a broad look at trends
in inequalities in post-policy income over time and across countries. The
second takes snapshots at particular points in time to compare the magnitude of inequalities in market income (pre-policy) and in disposable
income (post-policy). Both types of analyses suggest that government policies have major effects on the magnitude of socio-economic inequalities.

Income inequalities over time and across countries

The 1950s to the late 1970s saw a convergence in the economic and social policies of high-income countries, with governments promoting high
employment and investing in welfare services. In consequence, inequalities in disposable income narrowed, a trend evident in the UK through
the 1950s. These decades also 'saw the US government transformed from
a traditional defense-transportation-natural resources enterprise to a major engine for poverty reduction' (Sefton, 2006: 617). Here, too, the share
of national income going to richer households fell (Mishel et al., 2006).
In countries which intervened most actively in the labour market and
invested most heavily in progressive and universal welfare systems, like
Finland, Norway and Sweden, income inequalities reached particularly
low levels (Atkinson et al., 1995).

From the late 1970s, policies in high-income countries started to di-
verge, with the UK leading the way. Its right-wing government saw state
intervention in the market and high levels of social expenditure as fetter-
ing economic growth and wealth creation. Across the 1980s and 1990s,
it therefore favoured deregulation of the market economy, reductions in

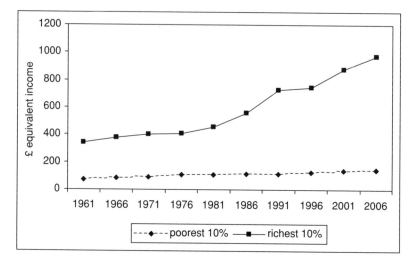

Figure 3.2.1 Weekly disposable income of the poorest and richest 10 per cent of households, before housing costs, 1961–2006.
Source: IFS (2008).

the progressiveness of taxation and cuts in public expenditure. Figure 3.2.1 captures the impact on income inequalities by focusing the weekly disposable incomes of the poorest tenth and the richest tenth of households. It suggests that the period of greater equality of income had come to an end by the early 1960s, and, while still marked, income inequalities remained stable through the 1960s and 1970s. From the late 1970s, real incomes at the upper end of the income distribution began to increase rapidly while incomes at the bottom stagnated. Since the 1990s, inequalities in disposable income have widened further. A key reason is that the value of the cash benefits and tax credits on which poorer households rely has grown less quickly than average incomes, and the incomes of the richest households in particular (Brewer et al., 2008).

Countries adopting similar policies have also experienced a sharp rise in income inequalities. For example through the 1980s and 1990s, the USA and New Zealand adopted the neo-liberal approach of the British government and income inequalities rose steeply in both countries across these decades (Dalziel, 2002; Mishel et al., 2006). The pattern has been repeated through the 1990s and 2000s in the world's emerging economies. For example in Russia, the shift from a centrally planned to a market-based economy and the collapse of collectively funded welfare systems have been accompanied by a marked widening of income inequalities (Förster et al., 2005).

But widening income inequalities have not been the universal pattern. In Canada, poverty rates fell from the 1970s to the 1990s – but rose sharply in the USA (Zuberi, 2001). Through the 1990s, inequalities in disposable income increased from an already high level in the UK but remained low in Sweden, despite the country experiencing a deep recession and rising unemployment (Palme et al., 2003). The major explanation of these diverging patterns is differences in domestic policies. As an international review of income inequalities concluded, 'even in a globalized world, the distribution of income in a country remains very much a consequence of the domestic political, institutional and economic choices made by those individual countries' (Smeeding, 2002: 28).

Inequalities in market income and in disposable income

To understand how policy choices affect inequalities in income, researchers have turned to a second type of analysis. This examines the effect on income inequalities of two instruments of redistribution: direct taxes and welfare benefits. The effect is often assessed by comparing the proportion of the population in poverty before and after taxes are deducted and welfare benefits are received.

Figure 3.2.2 provides an example of this type of analysis. It makes clear that, without government intervention through the tax and benefits systems, a high proportion of households would be in poverty in all countries. While government intervention appreciably reduces poverty rates,

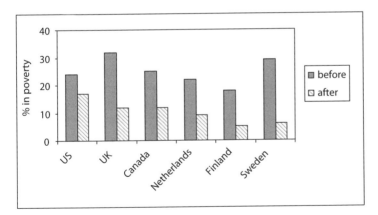

Figure 3.2.2 Poverty rates before and after income transfers (direct tax and welfare benefits), 2000.
Note: poverty defined as below 50 per cent of median household income, adjusted for household size and composition.
Source: adapted from Smeeding (2005), Figure 2.

the effectiveness of their intervention varies. Direct taxes and welfare benefits combine to reduce poverty rates in the USA from 24 per cent to 17 per cent (a reduction of 29%), and in the UK, from 32 per cent to 12 per cent (63% reduction). In Sweden, the poverty rate falls from 29 per cent to 6 per cent (79% reduction). A similar picture emerges from analyses focused on childhood, a period of life when disadvantaged circumstances have powerful effects on social and health trajectories (Chapter 1.1). While tax and benefit policies in Nordic countries lift a large proportion of children out of poverty, in the UK and USA, the policies are much less effective (Whiteford and Adema, 2006). The explanation lies in the progressiveness of the Nordic tax system and its structure of universal cash benefits which lift more people out of poverty and protect them from major drops in income during periods of unemployment and illness. The UK has a less progressive tax system and relies more heavily on means-tested benefits set below the poverty line (Stewart, 2005). In other words, 'different levels and mixes of government spending on the poor have sizable effects on national poverty rates' (Smeeding et al., 2001: 174).

This brief review makes clear that market economies produce deep inequalities. Without government intervention, inequalities in people's living standards (in their disposable incomes) would be as extreme as the inequalities in their market incomes; levels of poverty would also be very high. Deep inequalities and high rates of poverty would be particularly evident for economically dependent groups like children. But the taxation and welfare benefits systems provide powerful levers through which to temper these inequalities. Historical and comparative evidence suggests that, when governments are committed to reducing inequalities in people's socio-economic circumstances, they are successful: their policies lift incomes in poorer households and reduce incomes in richer households. When political commitment weakens, these policies become less redistributive. Taxation becomes less progressive and cash benefits are scaled back – and inequalities in living standards widen rapidly. As this indicates, the absence of a pro-equity policy is not neutral in its effects; instead, it fuels socio-economic inequalities.

Socio-economic inequalities in cigarette smoking: the scope for policy

A hundred years ago, death rates from coronary heart disease and lung cancer were low even in high-income countries in which the chronic disease epidemic first took hold. Today, these diseases are leading causes of death in high-income countries and, increasingly, across the world (Lopez et al., 2006).

Behind the changing patterns of disease lies the shift from agriculture-based economies to ones where manufacturing and service industries provide the engines of economic growth. The economic shift involves social changes too, with people moving to densely populated urban areas to work in factories and offices. The social changes, in turn, disrupt traditional food systems and long-established patterns of physical activity and tobacco use. Staple diets based on grains and vegetables give way to processed foods high in fats and sugars, manual work gives way to sedentary occupations, and traditional forms of tobacco use are replaced by manufactured cigarettes. This transformation of health-related behaviours has been identified as one of the major mechanisms through which economic change triggers changes in the patterns of disease (Graham, 2007).

Tobacco use provides an illustration. Until the 20th century, pipes, cigars, snuff and chewing tobacco were the dominant forms of tobacco use. Consumption was typically low and restricted to men (Wald and Nicolaides-Bouman, 1991; Brandt, 2007). The invention of manufactured cigarettes in the late 19th century transformed this traditional picture. The new product used a more palatable form of tobacco which was also more addictive. Produced by machine rather than by hand, cigarettes could be manufactured for the mass market which tobacco companies were quick to develop through advertising and other marketing strategies (Brandt, 2007). The result was a rapid increase in cigarette use, first among men and then among women.

In the UK for example, cigarette consumption among men increased markedly from 1900; by 1920 it had become the dominant form of tobacco use. Over the next two decades, consumption among women rose rapidly. The evidence suggests that men and women in privileged circumstances were the 'trendsetters', with the habit then spreading across the population. By the 1940s, over 65 per cent of men and 40 per cent of women in all socio-economic groups were cigarette smokers (Wald and Nicolaides-Bouman, 1991). Since then, rates of cigarette smoking have declined. However, the decline has been more marked among higher than lower socio-economic groups with the result that socio-economic gradients among both men and women have emerged and then steepened over time. At the same time, gender differences have narrowed. Figure 3.2.3 captures these trends by focusing on the highest socio-economic group (professional occupations) and lowest group (unskilled manual).

The patterns found in Britain are evident in the USA and in other northern European countries. Here, too, socio-economic gradients in smoking have emerged among men and women, with current trends suggesting that gradients will continue to steepen (Huisman et al., 2005; NCHS, 2007). Southern Europe is at an earlier stage of what has been called 'the cigarette epidemic' (Lopez et al., 1994). Smoking among women was rare

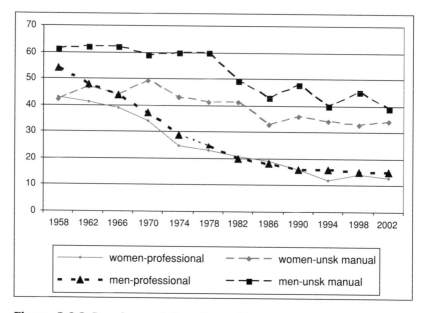

Figure 3.2.3 Prevalence of cigarette smoking among women and men in the highest (professional) and lowest (unskilled manual) socio-economic groups, Britain, 1958–2000.
Sources: Wald and Nicolaides-Bouman, 1991, table 5.2; Office for National Statistics, 2001, table 8.8.

until the closing decades of the 20th century: it was not until the 1970s in Italy, Spain and Greece, and the 1980s in Portugal, that women followed men into cigarette smoking (Graham, 1996). Again, there is evidence that trends have been led by younger and more affluent groups, with positive socio-economic gradients flattening over time. Among men, the association between socio-economic disadvantage and smoking remains less pronounced in Spain, Portugal and Greece than in northern European countries like the UK, Norway, Sweden and Denmark. Among women in these countries, smoking prevalence is still higher among women from more affluent backgrounds. However, the socio-economic gradients are flatter among younger age groups, presaging the emergence of the inequalities in smoking evident in northern Europe (Huisman et al., 2005). What is evident in Europe is now being repeated on a global scale. Through the early decades of the 21st century, the world's smoking population is set to become increasingly female and increasingly disadvantaged (Graham, 2009).

Smoking habits are typically established in adolescence, with most smokers taking up the habit in their teenage years. Because cigarettes dispense a highly additive drug, adolescent smoking can set in train a habit which persists into adulthood (Jefferis et al., 2003). Smoking careers are, in turn, shaped by people's socio-economic circumstances. A privileged journey through life – an advantaged childhood, success in the educational system and a place in the higher echelons of the occupational structure – is associated with lower rates of smoking and higher rates of quitting. Conversely, disadvantage pathways increase the risk of becoming and remaining a smoker. Among women, early parenthood is often part of these disadvantaged pathways, and contributes to the risk of being a smoker in adulthood (Graham et al., 2006).

Table 3.2.1 is based on the UK's *Millennium Cohort Study* which is following children born in 2000–1 (see Chapter 1.1 for details); when the children were 9 months old, 28 per cent of mothers smoked cigarettes. The table focuses on mothers from poorer childhood backgrounds, as measured by the UK's official socio-economic classification (see Hilary Graham's introductory chapter for details) among whom 33 per cent were smokers. It then looks within this group at mothers who had left school at or before the UK's minimum school-leaving age. In this group, smoking prevalence climbs to 44 per cent. It rises again to 63 per cent among the group who

Table 3.2.1 Disadvantaged trajectories and smoking status of mothers at nine months post-partum in the *UK Millennium Cohort Study*, 2001–2

	Number	Current smoker* (%)
All mothers	13573	28
Mothers with:		
childhood disadvantage[1]	6244	33
plus left full-time education ≤ 16	3464	44
plus a mother < 20	1059	63
plus adult disadvantage[2]	554	69
Mothers experiencing none of these disadvantages	3174	13

Notes: percentages weighted to take account of over-sampling of mothers from poorer areas and from areas with higher proportions of people from minority ethnic groups.

*≥ 1 cigarette a day.

[1] childhood disadvantage measured by father's occupation when the mother was aged 14 (routine and manual occupation, never worked, long-term unemployed).

[2] adult disadvantage defined as an annual household income of £11000 or less.

Source: Sherburne Hawkins, Graham and Law: unpublished analysis of *Millennium Cohort Study*.

also became mothers before the age of 20. For women who had faced these multiple disadvantages and whose current circumstances were also poor, prevalence was 69 per cent. In contrast, among those who had had none of these experiences, prevalence stood at 13 per cent.

How might policies influence the inequalities in cigarette smoking captured in Table 3.2.1 and the wider trends described in Figure 3.2.3? We know from evaluations of tobacco control interventions that there are effective ways of reducing overall levels of smoking. For example, interventions backed by government regulation (like price increases, clean indoor air laws, and comprehensive bans on advertising and promotion) and by government investment (consumer information, media campaigns, smoking-cessation services) are associated with reductions in overall tobacco use. We also know that the effectiveness of these measures tends to be greater when they form part of a comprehensive, well-funded strategy (Levy et al., 2004). However, because evaluations typically focus on the population level, they say little about the impact of tobacco control interventions on *inequalities* in smoking. With limited evidence to draw on, conclusions must be tentative and provisional. Four broad points can however be made.

First, there is considerable evidence that weak tobacco control policies are linked to widening inequalities in smoking. For example, while aware of the health risks of cigarette smoking by the early 1950s, the UK government's response across the decade was characterized by 'lack of action' and 'equivocal messages' (Berridge and Loughlin, 2005: 957). It was not until the 1960s that a voluntary ban was negotiated with the tobacco industry on television advertising before 9 pm, and it was the 1970s before government-funded television campaigns began to warn of the dangers of cigarette smoking (Berridge and Loughlin, 2005). Across these decades, socio-economic differentials in cigarette use widened rapidly (Figure 3.2.3). Evidence on specific tobacco control measures confirms the link between weak tobacco control policies and widening social inequalities in cigarette smoking. For example, weak controls on cigarette advertising are associated with increases in cigarette use among young people, and particularly among those on disadvantaged trajectories (see, for example, Pierce et al., 1998). Evidence from middle-income and low-income countries also suggests that, when the promotional activities of transnational tobacco companies go unchecked, smoking prevalence increases and does so particularly among economically vulnerable groups (see, for example, Lee et al., 2004). Putting this range of evidence together, we can conclude that socio-economic inequalities in smoking are likely to widen in the absence of strong and co-ordinated tobacco control policies.

Second, there is some evidence that strong tobacco control policies are associated with reductions in smoking in both advantaged and disadvantaged groups. This has been reported for young people, with effects which are at least as marked among more and less advantaged groups (Kim and Clark, 2006; White et al., 2008). A review of the impact of tobacco control policies on cessation rates among adults not only found that quit rates were higher in countries with stronger and more comprehensive polices; it found, too, that these beneficial effects were similar across socio-economic groups (Schaap et al., 2008). These are important findings. Because smoking rates are higher in poorer groups, a policy with the same magnitude of effect on all socio-economic groups (helping 1 in 100 smokers in all groups to quit, for example) would narrow the gap in smoking rates.

However, the positive effects of national policies will be blunted if they are not supported by a broader trans-national strategy (Collin, 2002). Because cigarettes are a global commodity – they are traded, marketed and smuggled across national boundaries – national policies can be easily undermined by 'global marketing, transnational tobacco advertising, promotion and sponsorship, and the international movement of contraband and counterfeit cigarettes' (WHO, 2003: v). It was for this reason that the WHO negotiated a global Framework Convention on Tobacco Control (FCTC). The global policy framework, which came into force in 2005, seeks to control tobacco advertising, promotion and sponsorship, the packaging and labelling of cigarettes, and the illicit trade in tobacco products as well as protecting people from exposure to second-hand smoke. It is too early to tell whether it will halt the trend towards widening socio-economic inequalities in tobacco use within countries and across the world.

A third point is relevant here. While tobacco control policies have an important contribution to make to narrowing socio-economic inequalities in tobacco use, their impact is likely to be modest. An European analysis found that, even countries which had introduced the most effective policies, marked socio-economic gradients in smoking remained (Schaap et al., 2008). As in other international analyses, the UK scored highly with respect to the strength of its tobacco control policies. While it is too soon for analyses to measure the effects of recent UK interventions (like legislation requiring that indoor public spaces are smoke-free), tobacco control policies would need to achieve a magnitude of effect far beyond that achieved to date if they were to eliminate inequalities in smoking. The persisting gradients in smoking captured in Figure 3.2.3 point to the importance of policies which address 'the causes of the causes': the social factors which leave poorer groups at greater risk of taking up cigarette smoking in adolescence and remaining a smoker in later life (see Table 3.2.1).

This leads to a fourth conclusion. An equity-oriented approach needs to include not only interventions focused on tobacco use. It also requires policies which address inequalities in people's lives. As evidence from the

UK suggests, tackling widening inequalities in cigarette use (Figure 3.2.3) is likely to be an uphill task when broader socio-economic inequalities are widening (Figure 3.2.1) and when key policy levers like fiscal and welfare policies are leaving a large proportion of the population in poverty (Figure 3.2.2). It is a conclusion underlined by studies of smokers in disadvantaged circumstances. The studies make clear that the motivation and self-efficacy needed to quit are easier to mobilize in communities who can see their lives are improving and the prospects for their children are looking brighter (Dorsett and Marsh, 1998). Conversely, even well-designed and well-delivered interventions will struggle to reduce smoking in communities whose lives are blighted by chronic hardship and where few expect the future to be better (Dorsett and Marsh, 1998; Wiltshire et al., 2003).

Conclusion

Tackling socio-economic inequalities in health has become a central goal of public health policies at national and international levels. According to the policy blueprints, the goal can be achieved by tackling the wider determinants of health. To be effective, such an approach needs to level up access to health determinants across socio-economic groups. The chapter has examined how policies can do this by focusing on inequalities in socio-economic circumstances (living standards) and health behaviour (cigarette smoking). Common themes emerge.

For both determinants, there is convincing evidence that their distribution becomes more unequal in the absence of government intervention. Doing nothing does not mean that nothing happens. Instead, inequalities in living standards and cigarette smoking widen without strong pro-equity policies. Thus, when governments retreat from progressive taxation and welfare policies, inequalities in income increase rapidly; in the absence of strong universal policies for tobacco control, inequalities in cigarette smoking have also widened rapidly.

This leads onto another common theme: government intervention in market economies holds the key to moderating inequalities in health determinants. For example, progressive policies for taxation and welfare benefits temper market-generated inequalities in income, leaving households much less unequal and poverty rates much lower than they would otherwise be. There is increasing evidence, too, that policies which regulate the tobacco industry – for example, by controlling the production, marketing, price, purchase and consumption of cigarettes – may be effective among both advantaged and disadvantaged groups. For both determinants therefore, strong governance structures are central to tackling health inequalities. Through the 1980s and 1990s, powerful countries like the USA and powerful international agencies like the World Bank and the International Monetary Fund rejected market regulation and government intervention. The global economic recession triggered in 2008 by the collapse of this free-market doctrine leaves their approach in tatters. There is therefore a real opportunity to develop regulatory institutions and interventionist policies which are 'equity proofed' and therefore pro-poor.

A final common theme emerges: policy synergies are important. The effectiveness of an individual intervention may be conditional on other policies being in place: for example, equity-oriented social policies may be a precondition for progress in reducing inequalities in smoking. Conversely, when policies are combined – for example, when effective tobacco control interventions form part of a comprehensive strategy and when progressive policies on taxation and welfare benefits are pursued in tandem – their effects can be substantial. As this suggests, there is indeed scope for policies to reduce health inequalities – and without strong equity-oriented policies, inequalities are set to widen.

Note

1. In most high-income countries, 'welfare' is used to describe the range of benefits and services which enable people to 'fare well' through their lives. In the USA, 'welfare' has a narrower meaning. It typically describes one particular cash benefit, Aid to Families with Dependent Children (AFDC), which was replaced in the mid-1990s by a welfare-to-work programme, called Temporary Assistance for Needy Families (TANF).

Acknowledgements

The unpublished analyses of the Millennium Cohort Study in Table 3.2.1 were undertaken with Summer Hawkins and Catherine Law, UCL Institute of Child Health, London.

References

Advisory Committee on Population Health and Health Security (ACPHHS) (2005) *The Integrated Pan-Canadian Healthy Living Strategy*. Ottawa: Public Health Agency of Canada.
Ågren, G. (2003) *Sweden's New Public Health Policy*. Stockholm: National Institute for Public Health.

Amenta, E. and Skocpol, T. (1989) Explaining the distinctiveness of American public policy in the last century, in F.G. Castles (ed.) *The Comparative History of Public Policy.* Cambridge: Polity Press.

Atkinson, A.B., Rainwater, L. and Smeeding, T.M. (1995) *Income Distribution in OECD Countries,* Social Policy Studies No. 18. Paris: Organization for Economic Co-operation and Development.

Beaglehole, R. and Magnus, P. (2002) The search for new risk factors for coronary heart disease: occupational therapy for epidemiologists? *International Journal of Epidemiology,* 31: 111–22.

Berridge, V. and Loughlin, K. (2005) Smoking and the new health education in Britain, 1950s–1970s, *American Journal of Public Health,* 95(6): 956–64.

Brandt, A.M. (2007) *The Cigarette Century.* New York: Basic Books.

Brewer, M., Muriel, A., Phillips, D. and Sibieta, L. (2008) *Poverty and Inequality in the UK: 2008.* London: Institute for Fiscal Studies.

Collin, J., Lee, K. and Bissell, K. (2002) The framework convention on tobacco control: the politics of global health governance, *Third World Quarterly,* 23: 265–82.

Dalziel, P. (2002) New Zealand's economic reforms: an assessment, *Review of Political Economy,* 14(1): 31–46.

Department of Health (DH) (2001) *Tackling Health Inequalities: Consultation on a Plan for Delivery.* London: DH.

Department of Health (DH) (2003) *Tackling Health Inequalities: A Programme for Action.* London: DH.

Dorsett, R. and Marsh, A. (1998) *The Health Trap: Poverty, Smoking and Lone Parenthood.* London: Policy Studies Institute.

Falkingham, J. and Hills, J. (eds) (1995) *The Dynamic of Welfare: The Welfare State and the Life Cycle.* Hemel Hempstead: Prentice Hall/Harvester Wheatsheaf.

Förster, M., Jesuit, D. and Smeeding, T. (2005) Regional poverty and income inequality in Central and Eastern Europe, in R. Kanbur and A.J. Venables (eds) *Spatial Inequality and Development.* Oxford: Oxford University Press.

Ginsberg, N. (1993) Sweden: the social democratic case, in A. Cochrane and J. Clarhe (eds) *comparing Welfare States: Britain in International context.* Milton Keynes: The Open University.

Graham, H. (1996) Smoking prevalence among women in the European Community 1950–1990, *Social Science and Medicine,* 3: 242–47.

Graham, H. (2004) Social determinants and their unequal distribution: clarifying policy understandings, *Millbank Quarterly,* 82(1): 101–24.

Graham, H. (2007) *Unequal Lives: Health and Socioeconomic Inequalities.* Maidenhead: The Open University.

Graham, H. (2009) Women and smoking: *Drug and Alcohol Dependence.* doi:10.1016/f.drugalcdep.2009.02.009.

Graham, H., Francis, B., Inskip, H., Harman, J. and the SWS Study Team (2006) Socio-economic lifecourse influences on women's smoking status in early adulthood, *Journal of Epidemiology and Community Health,* 60: 228–33.

Graham, H. and Kelly, M.P. (2004) *Health Inequalities: Concepts, Frameworks and Policy.* Available at: http://www.nice. org.uk/aboutnice/whoweare/aboutthehda/evidencebase/keypapers/ papersthatinformandsupporttheevidencebase/health_inequalities_ concepts_frameworks_and_policy_briefing_paper.jsp.

Huisman, M., Kunst, A.E. and Mackenbach, J.P. (2005) Educational inequalities in smoking among men and women aged 16 years and older in 11 European countries, *Tobacco Control,* 14: 106–13.

Institute for Fiscal Studies (IFS). (2009) *Inequality, Poverty and Well-being Spreadsheet.* Available at: http://www.ifs.org.uk/projects_research. php?heading_id=8_

Jefferis, B.J., Graham, H., Manor, O., Power, C. (2003) Level of cigarette smoking and socio-economic circumstances in adolescence: how do they affect adult smoking? *Addiction,* 98: 1765–72.

Kim, H. and Clark P.I. (2006) Cigarette smoking transition in females of low socio-economic status: impact of state, school and individual factors, *Journal of Epidemiology and Community Health,* 60(suppl II): ii13–ii19.

Lee, K., Gilmore A.B. and Collin, J. (2004) Breaking and re-entering: British American Tobacco in China 1979–2000, *Tobacco Control,* 13(suppl II): ii88–ii95.

Levy, D.T., Chaloupka, F.J. and Gitchell, J. (2004) The effects of tobacco control policies on smoking rates: a tobacco control score card, *Journal of Public Health Management Practice,* 10: 338–53.

Lopez, A.D., Mathers, C.D., Ezzati, M., Jamison, D.T. and Murray, C.J.L. (2006) *Global Burden of Disease and Risk Factors.* Oxford: Oxford University Press and World Bank.

Minister of Health (MH) (2000) *The New Zealand Strategy.* Wellington: MH.

Ministry of Health and Social Affairs (MHSA) (2000) *Health on Equal Terms: National Goals for Public Health.* Stockholm: MHSA.

Mishel, L., Bernstein, J. and Allegretto, S. (2006) *The State of Working America, 2006–07.* Washington DC: Economic Policy Unit.

National Center for Health Statistics (NCHS) (2007) *Health, United States 2007.* Washington DC: US Government Printing Office.

Norwegian Ministry of Health and Care Services (NMHCS) (2007) *National Strategy to Reduce Social Inequalities in Health*. Oslo: NMHCS.

Palme, J., Bergmark, A., Backman, O. et al. (2003) A welfare balance sheet for the 1990s, *Scandinavian Journal of Public Health*, suppl, 6: 7–143.

Pierce, J. P., Choi, W.S., Gilpin, E.A., Farkas, A.J. and Berry, C.C. (1998) Tobacco industry promotion of cigarettes and adolescent smoking, *Journal of the American Medical Association*, 279: 511–15.

Schaap, M.M., Kunst, A.E. and Leinsalu, M. et al. (2008) Effect of nationwide tobacco control policies on smoking cessation in high and low educated groups in 18 European countries, *Tobacco Control*, 17: 248–55.

Secretary of State for Health (SSH) (1999) *Saving Lives: Our Healthier Nation*, Cm 4386. London: The Stationery Office.

Secretary of State for Scotland (SSS) (1998) *Working Together for a Healthier Scotland: A Consultation Document*. Cm 3584. Edinburgh: The Stationery Office.

Sefton T. (2002) *Recent Changes in the Distribution of the Social Wage*, CASE paper 62. London: Centre for Analysis of Social Exclusion.

Sefton, T. (2006) Distributive and redistributive policy, in M. Moran, M. Rein and R.E. Goodin (eds) *The Oxford Handbook of Public Policy*. Oxford: Oxford University Press.

Smeeding, T.M., Rainwater, L. and Burtless, G. (2001) US poverty in cross-national perspective, in S.H. Danziger and R.H. Haveman (eds) *Understanding Poverty*. Boston, MA: Harvard University Press.

Smeeding, T. (2002) *Globalization, Inequality and the Rich Countries of the G-20: Evidence from the Luxembourg Income Study (LIS)*. New York, NY: Maxwell School of Citizenship and Public Affairs, Syracuse University.

Smeeding, T. (2005) *Causes and Consequences of Social Vulnerability in Comparative Perspective: Luxembourg Income Study Working Paper no 417*. Luxembourg: LIS.

Stewart, K. (2005). Changes in poverty and inequality in the UK in an international context, in J. Hills and K. Stewart (eds.) *A More Equal Society? New Labour, Poverty, Inequality and Exclusion*. London: Policy Press.

Therborn, G (1989) 'Pillarization' and 'popular movements' two variations of welfare state capitalism: The Netherlands and Sweden, in F.G. Castles (ed.) *The Comparative History of Public Policy*. Cambridge: Polity Press.

United States Department of Health and Human Services (USDHHS) (2000) *Healthy People 2010*. Washington DC: USDHHS.

Wald, N. and Nicolaides-Bouman, A. (1991) *UK Tobacco Statistics*. Oxford: Oxford University Press.

White, V.M., Hayman, J. and Hill D.J. (2008) Can population-based tobacco-control policies change smoking behaviors of adolescents from all socio-economic groups? Findings from Australia: 1987–2005, *Cancer Causes Control*, 19: 631–40.

Whiteford, P. and Adema, W. (2006) *Combating Child Poverty in OECD Countries: Is Work the Answer?* DELSA/ELSA/WD/SEM(2006)7, OECD Directorate for Employment, Labour and Social Affairs. Paris: OECD.

Whitehead, M. and Dahlgren, G. (2007) *Concepts and Principles for Tackling Social Inequalities in Health: Levelling up Part I*. Copenhagen: WHO Europe.

Wiltshire, S., Bancroft, A., Parry, O. and Amos, A. (2003) 'I came back here and started smoking again': perceptions and experiences of quitting among disadvantaged smokers, *Health Education Journal*, 18(3): 292–303.

World Health Organization (WHO) (2003) *Framework Convention on Tobacco Control*. Geneva: WHO.

World Health Organization (WHO) (2005) *Bangkok Charter for Health Promotion in a Globalized World*. Geneva: WHO.

World Health Organization (WHO) (2008) Commission on Social Determinants of Health (CSDH) *Closing the Gap in a Generation: Health Equity Through Action on the Social Determinants of Health*. Geneva: Commission on Social Determinants of Health, WHO.

World Health Organization (WHO) Europe (1999) *HEALTH21: The Health For All Policy Framework for the WHO European Region*. Copenhagen: WHO Regional Office for Europe.

Zuberi, D. (2001) *Transfers Matter Most: Luxembourg Income Study Working Paper No 271*. Available at: www.lisproject.org/publications/liswps/271.pdf.

Index

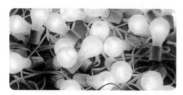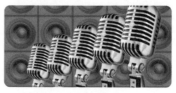
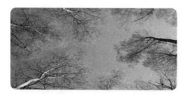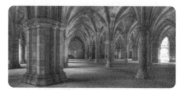
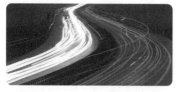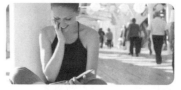
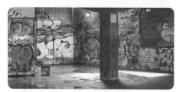
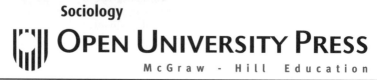